THE HUMAN SIDE OF MEDICAL TRAINING

Also in the series

Learning Under Pressure

THE HUMAN SIDE OF MEDICAL TRAINING

Studying for Medical School

Why Learning Feels Different and How to Adapt

Laura S. Woodward, Ph.D.

Threshold Academic Press

Royal Oak, Michigan

This book is for educational purposes only. It does not provide medical, psychological, or mental-health treatment, and it is not a substitute for professional care, academic advising, disability accommodations, or institutional guidance. The frameworks and examples are intended to support studying and learning under pressure. Readers experiencing persistent distress, health concerns, safety concerns, or academic difficulty beyond study strategy should seek qualified support from their institution or from an appropriate professional.

The information in this book reflects the author's experience and interpretation of research at the time of writing. Educational practices, institutional policies, and research findings may change over time.

This book was prepared with the assistance of artificial intelligence tools, under the author's direction, editing, and final review.

First edition.

ISBN: 979-8-9947927-4-2

Library of Congress Control Number: 2026915640

Printed in the United States of America

Threshold Academic Press

Royal Oak, Michigan

thresholdacademicpress@gmail.com

Start Here If You're Overwhelmed

You do not need to read this book cover to cover. Pick the sentence that sounds most like today, and start with that chapter.

I can't start. → Chapter 1 or 18

I study for hours and it's not sticking. → Chapter 4 or 5

I know it, then I blank. → Chapter 3 or 10

I'm anxious, or I'm avoiding. → Chapter 11 or 18

I feel behind everyone else. → Chapter 13 or 16

One bad week wrecked me. → Chapter 14 or 21

I'm exhausted. → Chapter 15

The environment is the problem. → Chapter 17

I doubt I belong here. → Chapter 12 or 19

Read ten pages. Pick one action. Stop.

One more thing, said plainly. This is a book about studying. It is not medical or mental-health care, and it is not meant to replace it. If what you are carrying runs deeper than study strategy, and it persists or touches your health or your safety, reaching for qualified support is the right move. Using help is part of doing this well.

Contents

INTRODUCTION

Studying Is Not a Character Test

Key Question

When studying stops working, what is the most useful question to ask first?

Core Idea

A missed question is information about the learning system, not a verdict on the learner.

A missed question can be read as a character problem (*the problem must be me*) or as a design problem. The second reading does not excuse the miss. It makes the miss usable by asking where the strain is coming from: load, access, strategy, emotion, recovery, or the systems the student is learning inside. Figure 1 illustrates the central distinction that runs throughout this book.

Load is the mental work a task asks of you at a given moment, and what happens when that work exceeds what working memory can manage. Access concerns retrieval: knowledge can be present and still remain hard to produce when a question calls for it. Strategy is the fit between a study method and the ability a task actually requires. Emotion covers the ways anxiety, self-doubt, and avoidance reach into learning itself.

FIGURE 1

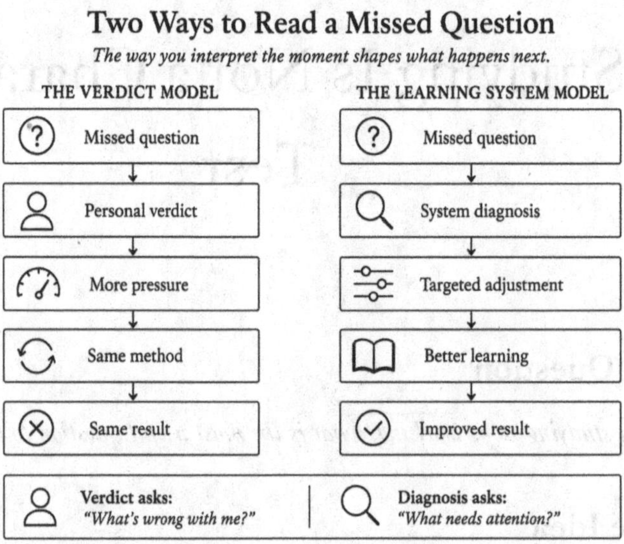

Figure 1. Two ways to read a missed question.

Recovery describes how sleep, stress, and fatigue limit what studying can accomplish. Systems are the training environments, evaluation structures, and culture that shape experiences which can otherwise feel entirely personal.

FIGURE 2

The Six Conditions of Learning

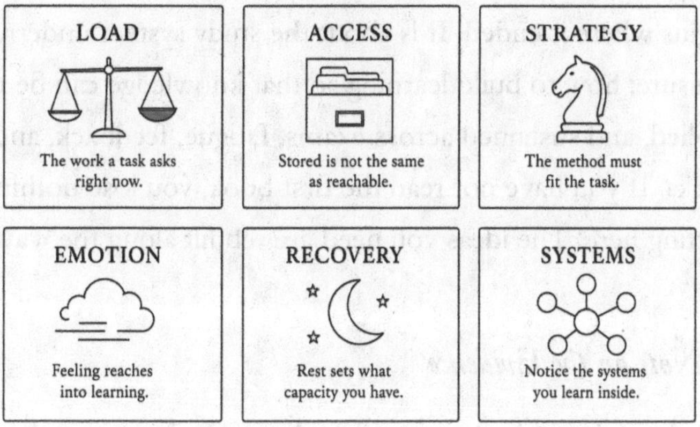

Figure 2. The six conditions of a learning system.

Figure 2 sets the six conditions side by side. Together they address a common problem in medical education. Students often evaluate themselves when the more useful move is to examine the conditions under which learning is occurring. When studying stops working, the question is usually not *What is wrong with me?* It is *What is happening in this learning system, and where is it breaking down?*

That shift does not make medical training easy. It does not remove the need for effort. It changes how struggle is interpreted, so that a setback does not become evidence about personal worth.

A learning system can be examined, adjusted, and improved. That is where this book begins.

If you are unsure where to start, the Start Here page at the front offers a route in, and the Field Manual at the back turns each condition into tools you can use in the middle of a hard week.

If you have read *Learning Under Pressure*, the first book in this series, parts of that frame will feel familiar, and that is by design. The earlier book is about why studying, recall, and performance change under pressure, and how to keep functioning when access drops. This one begins where it ended. It is about the study system underneath the pressure: how to build learning so that knowledge can be retrieved, applied, and sustained across exams, fatigue, feedback, and uneven weeks. If you have not read the first book, you lose nothing by starting here. The ideas you need are rebuilt along the way.

A Note on the Evidence

This book is not built on a single theory. It draws together several bodies of research: cognitive load theory, retrieval practice, metacognition, clinical reasoning, stress and recovery, self-regulated learning, student belonging, and the study of medical education systems. Where a specific claim rests on a specific study, the source is cited in the chapter where the claim appears.

PART ONE

Why Studying Breaks, and Why It's Not You

The Introduction made a single move: when studying stops working, the more useful question is what the learning system is asking of you. Part One stays with that question and narrows it. Before any method changes, it helps to see why learning breaks down in the first place.

Two conditions anchor the chapters that follow. The first is cognitive load, the mental work a task demands at a given moment. When that demand exceeds available capacity, studying becomes harder to start, harder to sustain, and less likely to produce useful learning.

The second is access, the ability to retrieve information when it is needed. Storing knowledge and reaching it under pressure are separate tasks, and much of the frustration in medical education comes from confusing familiarity with recall.

Two other questions complete this part of the book: how what you already know changes the weight of new material, and how to measure progress so that what gets counted is learning instead of activity. Together with load and access, these shape much of what feels like personal failure early in training. Naming them gives you a more accurate place to begin.

CHAPTER ONE

When Studying Asks More Than Your Mind Can Hold

Key Question

Why can studying feel impossible even when motivation is intact?

Core Idea

Studying breaks down when a task asks more of working memory than it can hold.

Example Scenario

Maya is a first-year medical student who likes structure. Before medical school, effort usually solved the problem. If a course felt difficult, she studied longer. If an exam went poorly, she adjusted her schedule, revised her plan, and worked harder.

Now she is doing all of those things, and the results no longer feel reliable. Her notes are color-coded, her calendar is organized, and her lecture recordings are marked with timestamps for review. Each adjustment feels responsible, but together they leave her increasingly exhausted.

As midnight approaches, Maya reaches a conclusion many medical students eventually reach: *maybe I am just not doing this well enough.* The conclusion feels personal because the struggle feels personal.

What Maya cannot easily see is that the problem may have less to do with commitment than with capacity: the amount of information, decision-making, and mental work her brain is being asked to manage at once. The more useful explanation is cognitive load.

Underneath what Maya feels as exhaustion, something quieter is at work. When a task asks for more than working memory can hold, the strain arrives as tiredness and self-doubt well before it announces itself as load, and one tired evening reveals the mechanism more than it reveals anything about her.

What Cognitive Load Means

Every act of studying depends on working memory. Working memory is the mental workspace used to hold information temporarily while thinking, comparing, reasoning, and making decisions.

Working memory is smaller than it feels like it should be. Only a small amount of information can be actively held and worked with at one time, and medical education places unusually heavy demands on that limited space (Cowan, 2001).

This idea has a name in the research: cognitive load theory, which explains why learning breaks down once the demands on working memory exceed what it can hold (Sweller, 1988). The same idea has since been applied directly to medical education, to explain how complex clinical material can overwhelm a learner and how instruction can be designed to avoid that (van Merriënboer & Sweller, 2010).

Some of the load comes from the material itself. Acid-base physiology places greater demands on working memory than memorizing a short list of medications. Some of the load comes from the way the task is organized, including unclear goals, multiple resources, disorganized notes, and vague instructions such as "review everything."

Studying becomes difficult when those demands accumulate faster than working memory can manage them. What looks like refusal is capacity running out: the brain is attempting to handle more information than it can process at that moment.

Why Overload Often Feels Personal

One reason cognitive overload is difficult to recognize is that it rarely feels like overload. More often, it feels emotional.

It can feel like procrastination when starting becomes difficult. It can feel like anxiety when the amount of work seems impossible to manage. It can feel like self-doubt when familiar study methods stop producing familiar results.

The frustration is real, and the anxiety is real. What is less obvious is that these experiences often emerge when cognitive demands exceed available capacity.

Stress can make the problem worse. Prolonged stress can change attention, memory, and the way the brain processes information (Sapolsky, 2004). That matters when students are already carrying uncertainty, sleep disruption, academic pressure, and fear of falling behind.

The experience feels personal because it is happening to you. The mechanism, however, is often broader than the individual student.

Why Medical Studying Overloads So Quickly

Medical education stacks demands rapidly. The content is complex, the volume is high, and the consequences feel important. At the same time, many study tasks remain surprisingly vague.

Students are told to review the block, know the material, and be prepared. Those instructions sound reasonable, but they do not provide a clear entry point. A learner facing a large, poorly defined task must first figure out how to approach it before meaningful studying can begin.

A tired student facing high-volume, poorly bounded work will often appear less capable than they actually are. Add long hours, emotional stakes, and concerns about falling behind, and working memory may already be strained before the first concept is processed.

From the inside, this can feel like laziness or avoidance. From the outside, it may be interpreted the same way. Both interpretations risk missing the mechanism.

Many study sessions become difficult before learning even begins. To start studying, Maya must decide what to work on, which resource to use, where to begin, how long to spend on it, and whether she is making the right choice.

Each decision requires mental effort. Taken individually, the decisions seem small. Together, they create a substantial burden.

This is the hidden cost of restarting. When tasks are large, vague, or poorly defined, the brain repeatedly returns to the same questions: *What should I study? Where do I start? How much is enough? Which resource should I trust?*

Every restart requires another round of decisions before academic work can begin. By the end of an evening, a surprising amount of mental energy may have been spent organizing the work instead of doing it.

Motivation often receives the blame in these situations. Capacity is frequently the more relevant issue. When a task feels too large, too vague, or too threatening to begin, avoidance becomes more likely. Pychyl and Sirois describe procrastination as closely tied to emotion regulation, which means avoidance may temporarily reduce distress even when it makes the larger problem harder to solve (Pychyl & Sirois, 2016). This does not mean avoidance is inevitable. It means the task may need redesign.

The Environment Around the Task

Cognitive load does not come only from the material and the way a task is organized. It also comes from what surrounds the task while you work.

A phone within reach is a standing example. Even face-down and silent, a phone can reduce the working memory available for the task in front of you, because part of attention stays in reserve for it whether or not you check it (Ward et al., 2017). The pull does not have to be answered to cost something.

Each interruption also carries the restart cost this chapter already described. Switching away and back does not resume cleanly. A residue of the previous task lingers and takes time to clear (Leroy, 2009). A glance that feels like seconds can cost far more in the reload that follows, and part of what students experience as fatigue comes from these repeated reloads.

The useful moves are environmental, because they spare capacity that is already under strain. Put distance between you and the phone, since out of the room tends to beat face-down on the desk. Close the loop before you start, with notifications off and the extra tabs closed, so the choice to switch is not offered mid-session. And when you are interrupted, leave a re-entry note of where you were, which makes the reload cheaper the way settling tomorrow's first task in advance does.

Why More Effort Can Make It Worse

The most common advice students receive when studying feels ineffective is to do more. More hours, more intensity, and more pressure can sound reasonable when the stakes are high.

Under conditions of overload, that advice can become counterproductive. Demanding more output from a depleted system often produces more depletion.

The more workable response is often load reduction. That means clarifying the task, shrinking the scope, reducing unnecessary demands, and protecting recovery.

When the burden on working memory returns to a manageable range, learning has a better chance to restart. Seriousness was never the missing piece. The fix is a task that allows effort to reach the work.

Redesigning the Task

Effective studying begins with reducing the cost of starting. The difference between a workable task and an unworkable task is often specificity.

"Review cardiology" leaves dozens of decisions unresolved.

"Complete fifteen flashcards on heart failure and sketch the Frank-Starling curve from memory" gives the brain a clear place to begin. The second task does not require more discipline. It requires fewer decisions, which allows cognitive energy to move toward learning instead of planning.

Psychologist Peter Gollwitzer's work on implementation intentions suggests that specific plans increase the likelihood that intended actions occur (Gollwitzer, 1999). The value of a plan is not simply organization. It removes decisions that would otherwise need to be made under conditions of fatigue.

The most useful adjustments are small ones that strip out decisions and lower the cost of the first action. They keep the standard in place and make it easier for effort to reach the work that matters.

What This Does Not Mean

Effort still matters. It just needs a task built well enough to receive it.

Try This Today

What to do: Choose one study task you have been avoiding. Rewrite it so that the first action is obvious and can be started immediately.

The pattern is the cardiology example above: an exact first action, small enough to start now.

What you may notice: The smaller task may feel unimpressive. It may even feel too easy, especially if you are used to treating large tasks as proof that you are taking the work seriously.

Why it matters: A task that feels too small but gets completed is usually more useful than a task that feels ambitious but never begins. Reducing the cost of starting creates conditions in which learning can occur.

Options Menu

Reducing load means finding the one place a task is asking too much and easing it there. Reach for whichever fits:

- **Shrink the task to an obvious first action.** Replace *review cardiology* with *fifteen flashcards on heart failure, then sketch the Frank-Starling curve from memory*. The smaller task can feel unserious, and it is the one that actually begins.

- **Decide tomorrow's first task before you stop tonight.** Settling the next action in advance spares you the cost of choosing while depleted, and specific plans of this kind make the intended action more likely to follow (Gollwitzer, 1999).

- **Limit open resources.** One primary source per topic, the extra tabs closed. You may feel you are missing something, and you stop paying the tax of switching between them.

- **Put the structure on paper instead of in your head.** A concept map, a class hierarchy, or a side-by-side chart carries organizing work that working memory would otherwise hold, and lowers the load the task places on it (Wong, 2015; van Merriënboer & Sweller, 2010).

Common Traps

A few responses to overload feel responsible and quietly deepen it.

Holding onto a large, vague task as proof of seriousness keeps the work hard to enter, so the evening's energy goes to deciding instead of learning, and the stall then looks like a problem of discipline.

Answering overload with more hours and more pressure assumes effort is the missing ingredient. Applied to a depleted system, it tends to produce more depletion. What the system needs is a task it can actually begin.

Keeping several resources open guards against missing something. Each switch reloads working memory from the start, and the reloads add up.

Recap

What to hold onto when studying will not start:

- **When a session is hard to begin**, look at the task before you look at your character.
- Cognitive load is the work a task asks of working memory right now, and overload often shows up disguised as procrastination, anxiety, or self-doubt.
- A large, vague task spends your energy on decisions before any learning starts.

- Under overload, more pressure usually deepens the problem, while a clearer, smaller task lets effort reach the work.

- Reducing load keeps the standard intact and gives effort a way to meet it.

Before You Move On

This chapter has focused on why studying becomes difficult to start. Sometimes the task is too large, too vague, or too decision-heavy for the learner's current capacity.

Load does not come only from the task. It also depends on what the new material can rest on. The same lecture can feel manageable to one student and crushing to another, and the difference is often what each already knows.

The next chapter looks at prior knowledge: why a thin foundation makes new material feel heavier than it is, and how to check the foundation before blaming the effort.

References

Cowan, N. (2001). The magical number 4 in short-term memory: A reconsideration of mental storage capacity. *Behavioral and Brain Sciences, 24*(1), 87–114.

Gollwitzer, P. M. (1999). Implementation intentions: Strong effects of simple plans. *American Psychologist, 54*(7), 493–503.

Leroy, S. (2009). Why is it so hard to do my work? The challenge of attention residue when switching between work tasks. *Organizational Behavior and Human Decision Processes, 109*(2), 168–181.

Pychyl, T. A., & Sirois, F. M. (2016). Procrastination, emotion regulation, and well-being. In F. M. Sirois & T. A. Pychyl (Eds.), *Procrastination, health, and well-being* (pp. 163–188). Academic Press.

Sapolsky, R. M. (2004). *Why zebras don't get ulcers* (3rd ed.). Holt.

Sweller, J. (1988). Cognitive load during problem solving: Effects on learning. *Cognitive Science, 12*(2), 257–285.

van Merriënboer, J. J. G., & Sweller, J. (2010). Cognitive load theory in health professional education: Design principles and strategies. *Medical Education, 44*(1), 85–93.

Ward, A. F., Duke, K., Gneezy, A., & Bos, M. W. (2017). Brain drain: The mere presence of one's own smartphone reduces available cognitive capacity. *Journal of the Association for Consumer Research, 2*(2), 140–154.

Wong, L. (2015). *Essential study skills* (8th ed.). Cengage Learning.

CHAPTER TWO

What You Already Know Sets the Ceiling

Key Question

Why does the same lecture feel manageable to one student and impossible to another?

Core Idea

New learning attaches to what you already know, so a gap in the foundation raises the cost of everything built on top of it.

Example Scenario

Nadia is three weeks into the renal block, and the diuretics will not stay put. She has watched the pharmacology lectures twice, made flashcards for every drug class, and reviewed them daily. Each card feels learnable on its own. Together they keep collapsing into a pile of syllables that could belong to any drug at all.

Her roommate covered the same material in two evenings and moved on. Watching that happen produces a familiar conclusion: *she is built for this, and apparently I am not.*

What Nadia cannot see from inside the block is what each of them brought into it. Her roommate took a renal physiology elective last spring. When a new drug arrives, it lands on a working model of the nephron, attaches to a transporter she can picture, and stays. For Nadia, each drug has nowhere to land, so each one must be memorized as an isolated fact and held there by force.

The difference between them is a foundation. Foundations are invisible from the outside, which is why the gap looks like talent.

Learning Is Not Built on Empty Ground

What happened to Nadia follows a general rule. Two students can attend the same lecture, read the same chapter, and leave with very different amounts of usable knowledge, and the difference often lies in what each already knew when the material arrived.

New information does not enter an empty space. It attaches to existing knowledge, and the strength of that existing structure shapes how easily the new material connects. When the foundation is solid, new detail has somewhere to land. When the foundation is thin, the same detail has nothing to attach to and must be held in isolation.

This is one of the most established findings in the study of learning. What a learner already knows is among the strongest influences on what they are able to learn next (Ausubel, 1968). It is also one of the least visible, because prior knowledge is silent. It shapes the experience without announcing itself.

Why a Thin Foundation Feels Like Overload

The previous chapter described cognitive load: the work a task asks of working memory in the moment. Prior knowledge is a large part of what sets that load.

When related knowledge is already organized in memory, a large amount of new information can be handled as a few familiar chunks. When it is not, each piece must be held separately, and working memory fills quickly. The same lecture is light for one student and overwhelming for another. The lecture did not change. The structures receiving it did.

This means overload is sometimes a foundations problem in disguise. A student drowning in a new block may not be failing to work hard enough or to manage load in the moment. They may be building on a base that cannot yet carry the weight, which makes every new concept more expensive than it should be.

Reading it this way changes the response. When the problem is a missing foundation, more hours spent on the current material produce diminishing returns, because the difficulty is upstream of where the effort is being spent.

The Foundations Question

Much of this book asks students to examine the conditions under which learning is occurring instead of their own character. Prior knowledge adds one more question to that check, alongside whether a task is overloaded, poorly designed, or badly timed: whether the base underneath it is solid enough to build on.

The question is there to locate the gap, and finding one carries no judgment. A foundations gap is common, it is specific, and it points to a specific response: go back far enough to find where the structure is sound, then rebuild forward from there. Renal pharmacology that will not hold is often a nephron-physiology problem wearing a pharmacology costume.

Two Ways to Use Prior Knowledge on Purpose

Because prior knowledge is silent, it helps to make it active before studying instead of assuming it is present.

One method is to test before you study. Attempting questions on new material before learning it, and expecting to miss some, surfaces what the foundation is missing, and the failed attempt itself can improve the learning that follows (Kornell et al., 2009; Richland, Kornell, & Kao, 2009). This is the desirable-difficulty logic from later in the book applied to the start of a topic instead of the review of it (Bjork & Bjork, 2011).

The other is to build the frame first. Reading a brief overview before the detail, or spending two minutes writing what you already know about a topic before opening the resource, gives the incoming material a structure to attach to. A rough map, built early, lowers the cost of everything placed on it afterward.

Neither method adds much time. Both convert prior knowledge from a hidden variable into something a student can check and strengthen deliberately.

Try This Today

What to do: Before studying a new topic, spend three minutes attempting a few questions on it, expecting to miss some. Note which ones expose a gap in something earlier rather than in the new material itself.

What you may notice: Some of what feels like difficulty with the new topic is actually a soft spot in an earlier one. The new material often becomes easier once the earlier gap is named.

Why it matters: Testing before studying shows you where the foundation is thin, and the attempt itself strengthens the learning that follows.

Options Menu

Prior knowledge sets the cost of everything built on it. These moves make it visible. Reach for whichever fits:

- **Test before you study.** Attempt questions on new material first, expecting to miss some. It feels backward, and the misses show you where the foundation needs shoring (Kornell et al., 2009).

- **Check the layer below.** When a new topic will not hold, test the prerequisite before adding hours to the current one. It costs a detour, and it often finds the real gap.

- **Build the frame first.** Read a short overview before the detail, so incoming material has somewhere to attach. It delays the deep dive, and it lowers the load of everything after it.

- **Write what you already know.** Two minutes mapping current understanding before opening the resource. It feels unnecessary, and it turns silent prior knowledge into a structure you can see.

Common Traps

A few habits treat a foundations problem as something else.

Answering a foundations gap with more hours on the current topic assumes effort is being spent where the difficulty lives. When the gap is upstream, the added hours land below the leak, and the returns diminish.

Reading early overwhelm as a load-management failure stops one step short. Sometimes the task is genuinely overloaded. Sometimes the base is thin. The two call for different responses.

Skipping the overview to save time removes the frame the detail was meant to attach to. The minutes saved at the start are usually repaid, with interest, in material that will not stick.

Recap

What to hold onto when the same material is far harder for you than it seems it should be:

- **New learning attaches to existing knowledge**, so what you already know sets the ceiling on what you can learn next, and the ceiling moves as the foundation is rebuilt.
- **A thin foundation shows up as overload**, because each new piece has nothing to attach to.
- The foundations question, whether the base is solid enough to build on, is a diagnosis without a grade.

- Testing before studying and building the frame first make prior knowledge visible and strengthen it.

Before You Move On

This chapter looked underneath cognitive load to the knowledge that sets it: what you already know determines how heavy new material feels, and a thin foundation raises the cost of everything above it. The response to a foundations gap is to rebuild from where the structure is sound instead of spending more effort at the surface.

Foundations shape how much you can take in. A separate problem is reaching what you have already stored. The next chapter turns to that: why material you understand can vanish the moment a question asks for it, and why storage and access are not the same task.

References

Ausubel, D. P. (1968). *Educational psychology: A cognitive view.* Holt, Rinehart & Winston.

Bjork, E. L., & Bjork, R. A. (2011). Making things hard on yourself, but in a good way: Creating desirable difficulties to enhance learning. In M. A. Gernsbacher, R. W. Pew, L. M. Hough, & J. R. Pomerantz (Eds.), *Psychology and the real world: Essays illustrating fundamental contributions to society* (pp. 56–64). Worth.

Kornell, N., Hays, M. J., & Bjork, R. A. (2009). Unsuccessful retrieval attempts enhance subsequent learning. *Journal of Experimental Psychology: Learning, Memory, and Cognition, 35*(4), 989–998.

Richland, L. E., Kornell, N., & Kao, L. S. (2009). The pretesting effect: Do unsuccessful retrieval attempts enhance learning? *Journal of Experimental Psychology: Applied, 15*(3), 243–257.

CHAPTER THREE

Knowledge Is Not the Same as Access

Key Question

Why can material you understand vanish the moment a question appears?

Core Idea

Recognizing material in front of you is a different skill from retrieving it when it is gone.

Example Scenario

Diego has been studying this topic for three days. He reviewed the lecture, completed the flashcards, and watched the explanation video twice. By the end of the third night, the material looked familiar, the diagram made sense, and the explanation felt easier to follow.

Then a practice question presents the same concept inside a clinical vignette. Diego stares at the screen, recognizing pieces of the problem without being able to produce the answer.

As soon as he misses the question, a conclusion arrives: *I thought I knew this, so I guess I did not.* Many students make the same interpretation because the experience feels like evidence that learning never occurred.

A more precise interpretation is that retrieval failure and learning failure are not always the same problem. They have different causes, and they require different responses.

One topic on one afternoon reveals little about everything Diego knows. The point is the pattern. The material was learned well enough to recognize, and not yet well enough to produce, and those two states call for different responses.

Storage and Retrieval Are Different Tasks

Learning depends on at least two processes that are easy to collapse into one. The first is storage, which means information has been encoded and retained in long-term memory. The second is retrieval, which means that information can be accessed when it is needed.

Much of what students call studying is designed to increase exposure. Re-reading, highlighting, reviewing notes, and watching explanations can make material feel familiar. Familiarity can be useful, especially when a student is first trying to understand a concept.

The problem begins when familiarity becomes the measure of preparedness. A concept can feel recognizable when it is in front of you and still be difficult to produce when a question requires it.

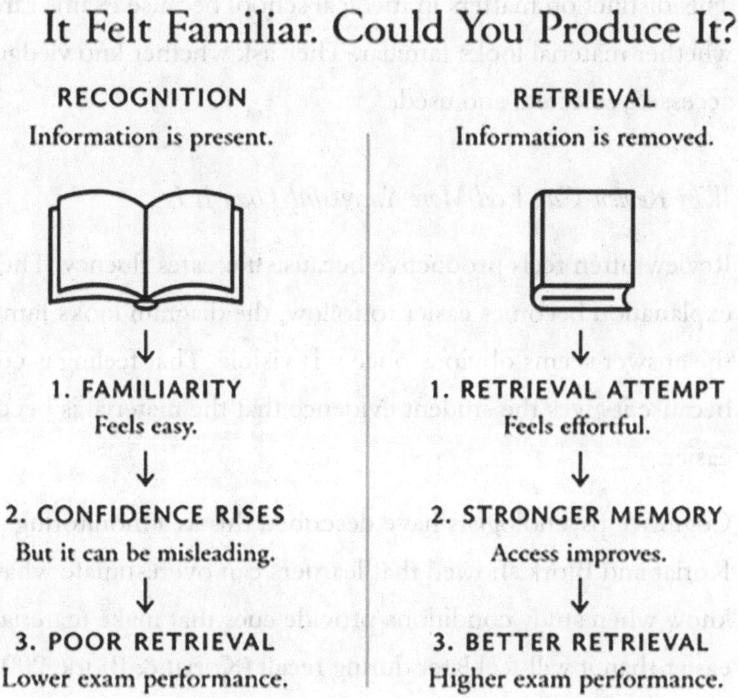

Figure 3. Review can create familiarity without strengthening retrieval.

Figure 3 draws this out. While the material sits in front of you, recognition rises and the answer feels available. Once it is gone, what remains is whatever you can retrieve on your own, which is the ability an exam measures.

Research on retrieval practice has shown that reviewing information and retrieving information are related but distinct learning activities. Roediger and Karpicke's work on test-enhanced learning demonstrated that taking memory tests can improve long-term retention, even when testing feels less reassuring than additional review (Roediger & Karpicke, 2006).

This distinction matters in medical school because exams rarely ask whether material looks familiar. They ask whether knowledge can be accessed, selected, and used.

Why Review Can Feel More Successful Than It Is

Review often feels productive because it creates fluency. The explanation becomes easier to follow, the diagram looks familiar, and the answer seems obvious once it is visible. That feeling is convincing because it gives the student evidence that the material is becoming easier.

Cognitive psychologists have described this as a monitoring problem. Koriat and Bjork showed that learners can overestimate what they know when study conditions provide cues that make material feel easier than it will feel later during recall (Koriat & Bjork, 2005).

Figure 4 traces the loop this sets up. Review builds recognition, recognition feels like confidence, and confidence quietly lowers the urge to test yourself. The gap stays hidden until a question asks for something you cannot produce. The way out is to trade some of the review for retrieval.

For Diego, this is exactly what happened. During review, the notes gave him cues. The headings, diagrams, and surrounding explanations helped the answer feel available. The question bank removed those cues and required him to generate the answer under different conditions.

Nothing mysterious happened when the practice question appeared. The task changed. Review asked Diego to recognize the material, while the question asked him to retrieve and use it.

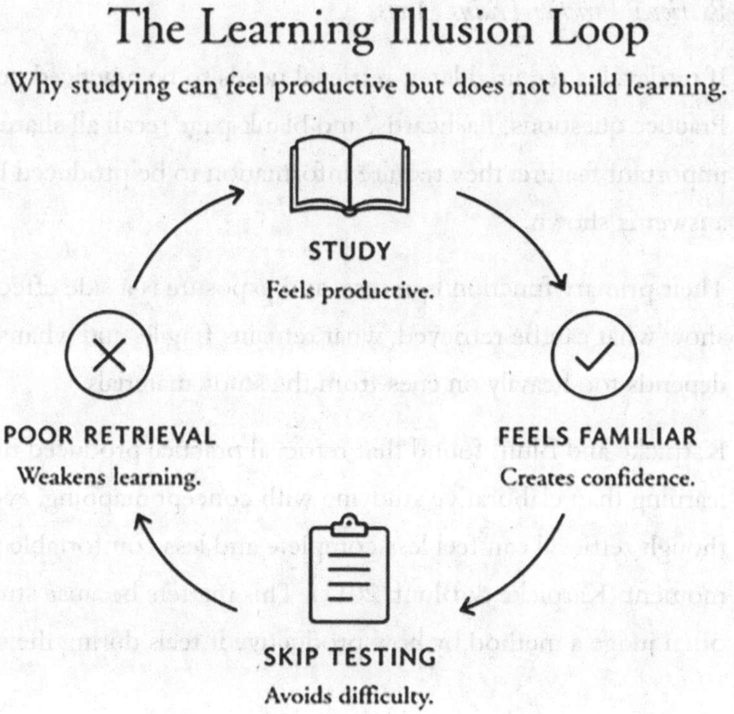

Figure 4. The learning illusion loop: review builds a feeling of progress without testing access.

The Retrieval Failure You May Be Misreading

When students blank on a question, they often assume the material was never learned, and reread it. Rereading helps when a concept was never understood, but the problem is frequently access: material reviewed at a desk, untimed, with the notes nearby is reached under very different conditions than a timed question set allows.

A retrieval failure can feel like a verdict. It reads more accurately as diagnostic information, less *Did I know this?* than *What made this hard to access?*

Retrieval Practice Trains Access

If retrieval is required later, retrieval needs to be practiced now. Practice questions, flashcards, and blank-page recall all share one important feature: they require information to be produced before the answer is shown.

Their primary function is access, and exposure is a side effect. They show what can be retrieved, what remains fragile, and what still depends too heavily on cues from the study materials.

Karpicke and Blunt found that retrieval practice produced more learning than elaborative studying with concept mapping, even though retrieval can feel less complete and less comfortable in the moment (Karpicke & Blunt, 2011). This matters because students often judge a method by how productive it feels during the session.

Why Retrieval Feels Worse Before It Works Better

One of the hardest parts of retrieval practice is that it can make students feel less confident at first. A review session may feel smooth, while a retrieval session may feel uneven, slow, and full of errors.

Robert Bjork and Elizabeth Bjork have described this kind of challenge as a desirable difficulty, meaning a difficulty that can slow performance during practice while supporting stronger learning later (Bjork & Bjork, 2011). The key is that the difficulty must serve learning.

This distinction matters for students like Diego. If he judges the session by how fluent it feels, review will seem superior. If he judges the session by whether it trains access, retrieval practice becomes more valuable.

A method can feel less successful in the moment while doing better work for later performance.

Four Reasons Retrieval Fails

When a question goes poorly, four different problems can produce the same outcome. The material was never encoded clearly enough. The material is stored but difficult to access under pressure. The concept is familiar while the question format remains unfamiliar. Or working memory was overloaded by fatigue, anxiety, or competing demands.

These problems look similar from the outside because they all produce a missed question. They do not require the same response.

If the material was never understood, the next step may be explanation. If the material was understood but inaccessible, the next step may be retrieval practice. If the question format was unfamiliar, the next step may be more practice with similar applications. If fatigue or anxiety interfered, the next step may involve changing the conditions under which studying or testing is happening.

Treating every missed question as proof that you need more review often misses the actual problem. The useful question is what kind of failure occurred. Slowing down long enough to answer it usually replaces a vague plan to "study more" with a specific next move.

A Question Is a Sample, Not a Verdict

Students often assume that every missed question reveals something global about their competence. A pharmacology question becomes evidence that they do not understand pharmacology. A difficult cardiology block becomes evidence that they are falling behind. The conclusion feels reasonable because performance is visible while competence is not.

Medical education researchers have repeatedly shown that performance varies substantially across cases, contexts, and question formats (Norman, 2005; Norman et al., 2006). Competence is not a single fixed quantity that reveals itself equally in every situation. Instead, examinations sample performance under specific conditions.

Missed questions still matter. The work is to read them accurately, as one of the kinds of failure named earlier instead of a verdict on ability.

The more useful question is what this particular result suggests about the conditions your learning is happening under right now. Competence is more than one question can measure.

Next action: after your next missed question, identify the most likely mechanism before deciding what to study next.

Try This Today

What to do: Choose one dense topic and build the single page you would want with you in the exam. Build it from memory first. Write down what you can produce without looking, and open your notes only afterward, to fill what is missing.

What you may notice: Deciding what belongs on the page takes more effort than rereading, and the gaps show themselves right away. By the time the page is finished, you often find you can do without it.

Why it matters: Choosing what matters and producing it from memory is retrieval practice. The finished page is a byproduct. The value lies in the work of making it, which rehearses the skill an exam asks for: reaching the knowledge once the material is closed.

Options Menu

There are several ways to train access, and each one asks you to produce information before any answer appears, which is the feature that strengthens later recall (Roediger & Karpicke, 2006). Choose whichever suits the topic:

- **Blank-page recall.** Close your notes, set two minutes, and write everything you can about a familiar topic, then compare it against the source. The gap is often wider than expected, and that gap is the information you came for.
- **Practice questions under exam conditions.** Work timed, without notes, in application formats. The conditions feel harsher, and they measure access the way the exam will.
- **Flashcards that ask for production.** Answer aloud or on paper before turning the card. Confirming that an answer looks right is review, and generating it first is retrieval.
- **Closed-book teaching.** Explain the concept aloud, without notes, as though to a colleague. Vague reasoning surfaces quickly, which is what makes the exercise useful.
- **Delayed self-testing.** Return to a topic a day or two after studying it, once some forgetting has set in. It feels harder, and that effort is part of why the retrieval holds.

Common Traps

A few habits feel like studying while training something other than access.

Rereading until the material feels smooth is reassuring, because smoothness reads as progress. The smoothness comes from familiarity, and familiarity fades the moment the notes close and a question asks you to produce the answer yourself.

Judging a session by how fluent it felt rewards the calm of review over the friction of retrieval. Retrieval almost always feels worse while it does more, so the session that exposes the most gaps is often the one that helped.

Reading every missed question as proof the material was never learned sends you back to reread what was already understood. The more useful move is to ask what kind of failure occurred, since a retrieval gap and a knowledge gap call for different responses.

Recap

What to hold onto when a question goes blank:

- Storing knowledge and reaching it under pressure are separate achievements, and the exam tests the second.
- **Familiarity grows whenever the page is open,** while access is the separate ability to produce the material once it closes.
- Retrieval practice feels worse than review because it shows you the gaps, and that exposure is the reason to do it.
- **A missed question is information about conditions**, so ask what kind of failure it was before deciding what to study.

- **When the exam asks for retrieval**, studying has to rehearse retrieval.

Before You Move On

Diego's mistake was not that he cared too little or studied too briefly. His mistake was using familiarity as evidence of access. Medical exams ask whether you can produce and use knowledge when the answer is no longer in front of you.

That distinction changes how studying should be designed. It also raises the next problem: if the methods that build access often feel slower and less reassuring, how should students measure whether studying is working?

That is where the next chapter begins.

References

Bjork, E. L., & Bjork, R. A. (2011). Making things hard on yourself, but in a good way: Creating desirable difficulties to enhance learning. In M. A. Gernsbacher, R. W. Pew, L. M. Hough, & J. R. Pomerantz (Eds.), *Psychology and the real world: Essays illustrating fundamental contributions to society* (pp. 56–64). Worth.

Karpicke, J. D., & Blunt, J. R. (2011). Retrieval practice produces more learning than elaborative studying with concept mapping. *Science, 331*(6018), 772–775.

Koriat, A., & Bjork, R. A. (2005). Illusions of competence in monitoring one's own knowledge during study. *Journal of Experimental Psychology: Learning, Memory, and Cognition, 31*(2), 187–194.

Norman, G. (2005). Research in clinical reasoning: Past history and current trends. *Medical Education, 39*(4), 418–427.

Norman, G., Bordage, G., Page, G., & Keane, D. (2006). How specific is case specificity? *Medical Education, 40*(7), 618–623.

Roediger, H. L., III, & Karpicke, J. D. (2006). Test-enhanced learning: Taking memory tests improves long-term retention. *Psychological Science, 17*(3), 249–255.

CHAPTER FOUR

Time on Task Is the Wrong Way to Measure Progress

Key Question

Why can hours of studying produce so little durable learning?

Core Idea

Activity measures effort, and learning is better judged by what you can retrieve and use.

Example Scenario

Elena leaves the library feeling productive.

She has been studying for most of the day. She reviewed her notes, completed her flashcards, watched several lecture videos, and reorganized a study guide. By the time she packs her bag, she feels tired in a way that seems reassuring. The effort and the hours were substantial, and the fatigue feels like evidence that something important happened.

Three days later, she sits down with a set of practice questions and discovers that much of the material feels less secure than she expected. Concepts that seemed familiar now require effort to recall. Details she thought she knew are difficult to retrieve. The experience leaves her confused because it conflicts with what she thought the study session had accomplished.

A single day reveals little about how Elena studies, but it exposes the gap this chapter is about: the session that felt most productive and the learning it actually produced were two different things.

Why Effort Feels Like Evidence

Students need some way to judge whether studying is working. Because learning is largely invisible, they often rely on indicators that are easy to see.

Time is one of those indicators. Hours can be counted. Resources can be completed. Flashcards can be reviewed. Notes can be highlighted. By evening, students can point to concrete evidence that work occurred.

Fatigue becomes another indicator. A long day of studying often feels productive because it was demanding. The exhaustion seems proportional to the amount of learning that occurred. The harder the day felt, the easier it becomes to assume that meaningful progress was made.

These conclusions are understandable because effort and learning are related. Learning usually requires effort, attention, and time. The difficulty is that effort does not provide a direct measure of what was learned. A student can work extremely hard and still study inefficiently. Another student can study for fewer hours and retain more.

Effort matters. The trouble starts when effort and learning are treated as interchangeable.

Learning and Performance Are Different Things

One of the most important findings in the learning sciences is that performance during practice can be a poor indicator of long-term learning. Soderstrom and Bjork describe learning and performance as related but distinct processes. Performance reflects what can be demonstrated now, while learning reflects changes that remain available later (Soderstrom & Bjork, 2015).

The distinction matters because students experience performance immediately and learning only after some delay. During a study session, they can observe how smoothly material is reviewed, how many questions are answered correctly, and how confident they feel. Those experiences create an impression of progress.

The challenge is that immediate performance can sometimes be misleading. A student may perform well during a study session because the material is fresh, the notes are available, or the context provides helpful cues. Those conditions can support performance without guaranteeing that the information will remain accessible later.

Learning reveals itself differently. Learning becomes visible when information can still be retrieved after time has passed, when concepts can be explained without notes, and when knowledge can be applied in unfamiliar situations. Those tests often occur long after the study session has ended.

This difference helps explain why students are sometimes surprised by their own results. They assume that strong performance during studying predicts strong performance later. In many cases it does. In some cases it does not.

Why Easy Studying Feels Better

Easy studying often produces reassuring signals. The material becomes familiar, explanations seem clearer, and concepts feel increasingly obvious. Students often leave these sessions with a sense that they have mastered the material.

That feeling deserves some respect. Familiarity is not meaningless. Understanding often begins with repeated exposure, and concepts usually become easier to process as knowledge develops.

The difficulty arises when ease becomes the primary measure of learning. Chapter Three showed why: material can feel familiar simply because it has been encountered repeatedly, and a student may know the wording of the notes well while the idea itself stays out of reach once the notes close.

This is one reason students often trust study methods that produce immediate confidence. The confidence feels informative. Sometimes it is. Sometimes it reflects familiarity more than learning (Kornell & Bjork, 2009).

Why Difficult Sessions Are Easy to Misjudge

The opposite problem occurs when a study session feels difficult.

A retrieval session produces mistakes, a question set exposes gaps, and an attempt to explain from memory reveals uncertainty. Chapter Three explained the mechanism. What matters here is the reading.

Students frequently leave these sessions discouraged because the work felt worse than review. Confidence declined at exactly the moment the measurement got honest.

The immediate experience can be misleading. A difficult study session may reveal weaknesses because it is measuring learning more honestly. The discomfort comes from discovering what is not yet accessible, which is different from failing to learn.

This distinction becomes important because students naturally prefer methods that produce reassuring signals. The methods that feel most productive are not always the methods producing the strongest learning.

How the session felt is one signal. What the session revealed about the state of your learning is the better one.

The Problem With Counting Hours

Medical students often track studying using numbers that are easy to count. They count hours studied, flashcards completed, videos watched, questions answered, and resources finished.

Two kinds of measure sit beside each other here. Activity measures (hours, questions completed, videos watched, pages read) capture effort and are easy to count. Learning measures (retrieval, application, delayed recall, discrimination) capture change and resist faking. Doing more and learning more can come apart.

These numbers are useful because they capture behavior. They can help students maintain consistency, build routines, and monitor effort over time. Activity measures are often valuable because studying does require sustained work.

The limitation is that activity measures do not directly assess learning. Completing a resource tells you that the resource was completed. It does not tell you what knowledge became accessible as a result. Spending six hours studying tells you that six hours were spent. It does not tell you how effectively those hours were used.

None of this means dropping the habit of tracking hours and effort. It means holding those numbers for what they are, a record of activity, and letting learning be measured on its own terms.

Measuring Learning Instead

If time, effort, and confidence are imperfect indicators, what should students look for instead?

A useful starting point is to focus on what knowledge can do. Instead of asking how much studying occurred, students can ask what abilities have improved as a result of studying.

- Can I retrieve this information without looking at my notes?
- Can I explain this concept clearly in my own words?
- Can I apply this idea to a new question?
- Can I distinguish this diagnosis from similar alternatives?
- Can I still access this information after some time has passed?

These questions are often less comfortable than counting completed tasks because they expose uncertainty. At the same time, they provide information that is more closely connected to learning itself.

Activity measures can stay. The correction is where they sit: in a supporting role, underneath the outcome they help produce.

Calibration Instead of Assumption

Students often assume that a productive study session produced learning and that a frustrating study session did not. Those assumptions are understandable because they are based on immediate experience.

A sounder approach is calibration. Calibration means checking how well your sense of knowing matches what you can actually do. Instead of assuming that confidence reflects learning, students look for opportunities to test that assumption. Instead of assuming that difficulty reflects failure, students examine what the difficulty reveals.

This shift matters because studying produces many signals that are easy to misinterpret. Familiarity can look like mastery. Fluency can look like understanding. Fatigue can look like productivity. Confidence can look like competence.

Calibration asks a different question. Instead of asking *How did this study session feel?*, students ask *What can I now do that I could not do before?*

That question is harder to answer, but it provides information that is more useful for future learning.

It helps to be honest about what the surrounding culture rewards. Countable effort gets the reinforcement: hours logged, cards cleared, videos finished, a resource marked complete. Those numbers are easy to see, easy to compare with classmates, and satisfying at the end of a long day. The exam rewards something quieter and harder to display: whether you can retrieve, apply, and discriminate under time pressure, with the page closed. Chasing the visible number is a reasonable response to the signals a day actually provides. The work is to notice the gap and begin tracking the thing the exam will measure, even when it counts for less on the surface.

Try This Today

What to do: Study a topic as you normally would. Several hours later, close your notes and explain the topic from memory. If possible, answer a practice question or teach the concept aloud.

What you may notice: Your delayed performance may differ from your immediate impression of learning. Material that felt secure may be difficult to retrieve, while material that felt uncertain may be more accessible than expected.

Why it matters: Learning often reveals itself over time. Performance reveals itself immediately. Treating them as identical can lead students to trust signals that are less informative than they appear.

Options Menu

If activity is the easy signal and learning is the one that matters, the move is to change what you track. Depending on the topic, you might trade:

- **Hours studied for topics you can explain without notes.** Harder to log than time, and much closer to what the exam asks.

- **Cards reviewed for cards you answered before turning them over.** Slower per card, and it counts access instead of exposure.
- Resources finished for questions you can now reason through that defeated you last week. Less tidy than a checklist, and it records change.
- **Same-day confidence for next-day performance.** Judge a topic a day after studying it. The truer signal arrives slower, and that slower signal is the one that counts.

Common Traps

Some of the most trusted signals turn out to be the least reliable.

Reading fatigue as proof of progress treats a hard day as a productive one. Exhaustion measures how demanding a session felt, which can rise even when little became accessible.

Trusting a session because it felt smooth rewards the comfort of familiar material. That smoothness usually means the cues were present, and it tends to disappear the moment the cues do.

Counting completion as learning offers the reassurance of a finished list. Finishing a resource confirms the resource is finished, and says little about what you could produce without it.

Recap

What to hold onto when a study day is hard to read:

- **You feel performance immediately and see learning only later**, which is why the two are easy to confuse.

- **Fluent sessions feel productive and can leave fragile learning**, while difficult sessions feel discouraging and often measure learning more honestly.
- Hours, cards, and videos record effort rather than outcome.
- Ask what you can now do that you could not before: retrieve, explain, apply, discriminate, recall after a delay.
- A discouraging session usually carries information rather than a verdict.

Before You Move On

This chapter has focused on another challenge: the signals students use to judge whether studying is working.

Learning and performance are related, but the two come apart more often than students expect. Some study experiences feel highly productive while producing fragile learning. Other study experiences feel frustrating while producing durable learning.

That observation raises the next question: if learning is not always visible during practice, which difficulties are helping and which are simply in the way?

The next chapter draws that line, and shows why the most useful difficulties are designed on purpose instead of encountered by accident.

References

Kornell, N., & Bjork, R. A. (2009). A stability bias in human memory: Overestimating remembering and underestimating learning. *Journal of Experimental Psychology: General, 138*(4), 449–468.

Soderstrom, N. C., & Bjork, R. A. (2015). Learning versus performance: An integrative review. *Perspectives on Psychological Science, 10*(2), 176–199.

PART TWO

How Learning Actually Improves

Part One examined why studying breaks down. Cognitive load can exceed working-memory capacity. Retrieval can fail even when knowledge is stored. Long hours can accumulate without producing the kind of learning medical exams require.

Part Two turns from explanation to design.

The central question is no longer why studying fails. It is how learning improves when study methods match the demands of the task.

Accumulation treats studying as taking in more information. Alignment begins with a different question: what will you need to do with that information? Recall it. Explain it. Apply it. Reason with it under pressure. The answer helps determine the method.

When studying is not improving, it gives you a place to start, asking which part of the learning system is under strain (load, access, strategy, emotion, recovery, or systems) before anything changes. The chapters in this part take up strategy, the part most directly concerned with how learning improves.

That shift changes how study sessions are built. It changes which difficulties are worth keeping, which errors deserve attention, and what performance data can actually tell you about learning.

Chapter Five begins with a deceptively simple question: if effort matters, what kinds of difficulty strengthen learning, and which kinds simply create more strain?

CHAPTER FIVE

When the Right Method Feels Wrong

Key Question

Why does an effective method often feel worse than the one it replaces?

Core Idea

Methods that build durable learning often feel harder because they reveal what you have not yet mastered.

Example Scenario

Kwame has a problem that many medical students eventually encounter. He knows that retrieval practice is supposed to help learning, so he starts replacing some of his review sessions with practice questions and recall exercises.

Within a week, he becomes concerned.

The study sessions feel worse.

He misses questions he thought he should answer correctly. He discovers gaps in topics he believed he understood. Material that felt familiar during review suddenly feels uncertain when he tries to retrieve it from memory.

Kwame reaches a conclusion that feels reasonable: *this new approach is not working.*

The problem is that he may be measuring the wrong thing.

The details vary from student to student, but the misread is common. The new approach felt worse because it was finally exposing what review had kept hidden.

By this point in the book, we have already seen that familiarity is not the same as retrieval and that performance during studying is not always a reliable measure of learning. The next step is understanding why some study methods feel more difficult than others and why that difficulty sometimes strengthens learning instead of interfering with it.

The important word is sometimes.

Not all difficulty is useful. Some difficulty supports learning. Some difficulty only makes learning harder. Understanding the difference can prevent students from abandoning effective strategies and help them avoid forms of struggle that add effort without adding value.

Why Easy Studying Feels So Convincing

Students naturally prefer methods that create a sense of progress, and there is nothing wrong with wanting studying to feel productive. The difficulty, as the previous chapter showed, is that the feeling of progress and the reality of learning do not always move together. Rereading and review feel reassuring because familiarity grows, so students tend to trust the methods that produce immediate confidence. The study methods that produce the strongest long-term learning do not always provide those same signals (Dunlosky et al., 2013).

Not All Difficulty Is Helpful

Students sometimes hear that learning requires struggle and conclude that difficulty itself is inherently valuable. That interpretation creates problems because difficulty comes in many forms.

A student trying to study after sleeping four hours is experiencing difficulty. A student switching constantly between resources is experiencing difficulty. A student attempting to learn five new topics simultaneously is experiencing difficulty.

None of these challenges improve learning merely because they are difficult.

Chapter One described these situations as cognitive load problems. The learner's attention is being consumed by factors that compete with learning instead of supporting it. The effort is real, but the effort is being spent in the wrong place.

This distinction matters because medical students sometimes mistake suffering for progress. Long hours, exhaustion, confusion, and frustration can create a sense that serious work is occurring. Sometimes serious work is occurring. Sometimes the student is working under poor conditions, and that is the whole story.

Useful difficulty strengthens learning. Unnecessary difficulty consumes resources that learning requires.

The challenge is learning to tell the difference.

What Makes a Difficulty Useful

A useful difficulty requires learners to perform some aspect of the task they will eventually need to perform later.

Retrieval requires learners to access information without being shown the answer. Spacing requires learners to reconstruct knowledge after some forgetting has occurred. Interleaving requires learners to distinguish among similar concepts. Self-explanation requires learners to organize and connect ideas in ways that reveal gaps in understanding.

These activities feel more demanding because they require more cognitive work from the learner.

Robert and Elizabeth Bjork describe these challenges as desirable difficulties because they may reduce performance during practice while improving learning over longer periods (Bjork & Bjork, 2011).

The phrase is useful because it emphasizes two important ideas. First, the difficulty is intentional. Second, the difficulty serves learning. Making studying harder is never the aim. The aim is conditions that strengthen the abilities students will eventually need.

Spacing: Learning After Some Forgetting

Many students prefer to study a topic repeatedly in a short period. The approach feels efficient because the material becomes increasingly familiar. Confidence grows, and performance during review often improves rapidly.

The problem emerges later.

When material is reviewed again immediately, retrieval requires very little effort because the information is still highly accessible. Students may perform well during the session while learning relatively little about what will happen after time has passed.

Spacing changes the task. Instead of reviewing immediately, students return after some forgetting has occurred. Retrieval becomes more difficult because the information is no longer sitting close to the surface.

That difficulty can feel discouraging. Students often interpret forgetting as evidence that learning failed.

Research on spaced practice suggests a different interpretation. Returning to material after a delay creates opportunities to reconstruct knowledge, and that reconstruction can strengthen long-term retention (Cepeda et al., 2006).

The forgetting is only the setup. The retrieval that follows is what matters.

Interleaving: Learning to Distinguish

Medical students frequently study one topic at a time. They complete a set of cardiology questions, then move to pulmonology, then move to nephrology.

The structure feels organized because each topic remains separate. Students often perform well during practice because the context makes it obvious which type of problem they are solving.

Interleaving changes that experience. Instead of studying similar problems together, students alternate among different categories and concepts.

Performance during practice often declines because learners must repeatedly identify which concept applies before they can solve the problem. The task becomes less predictable and more demanding.

That added difficulty serves a purpose. Medical practice rarely announces which diagnosis is present before asking a clinician to reason through the problem. The challenge is telling the possibilities apart, which takes more than recall.

Research suggests that interleaving can improve this kind of discrimination (Rohrer & Taylor, 2007).

Self-Explanation: Making Thinking Visible

Students often discover weaknesses in their understanding when they attempt to explain a concept aloud.

The material seemed clear while reading. The lecture seemed clear while listening. The notes seemed clear while reviewing. Then the student tries to explain the concept from memory and discovers uncertainty.

This experience can feel discouraging because it exposes gaps that were previously hidden. At the same time, those gaps are precisely what make the exercise useful.

Chi and colleagues found that self-explanation improves understanding because it requires learners to actively work with ideas instead of only encountering them (Chi et al., 1994).

The difficulty comes from making thinking visible. Students must organize concepts, connect ideas, and identify places where understanding remains incomplete.

Those demands increase effort during the study session. They also create opportunities for deeper learning.

Productive Failure: Learning Before You Know the Answer

Many students assume that learning should look successful from the beginning. If confusion appears early, they conclude that the strategy is failing. Research on productive failure suggests a different possibility (Kapur, 2008).

When learners attempt to solve a problem before receiving formal instruction, they often struggle. Their initial solutions may be incomplete, inefficient, or entirely incorrect. From the learner's perspective, the experience can feel like failure.

The surprising finding is that this struggle can prepare students to learn more effectively once instruction arrives. Early attempts make important features of the problem visible and create a framework that helps later explanations make sense.

This does not mean confusion is automatically beneficial. Productive failure works when the difficulty is connected to the task being learned. There is no value in staying stuck. The value comes from engaging with the problem deeply enough that future explanations have somewhere to attach.

Many medical students encounter this naturally. A complex physiology concept often becomes easier to understand after wrestling with practice questions that expose what remains unclear.

Next action: before reviewing a new topic, spend five minutes trying to explain or solve it from your current understanding.

What All of These Have in Common

Spacing, interleaving, retrieval, self-explanation, and productive failure look different on the surface, but they share one feature: each asks the learner to practice an ability they will need later. The difficulty is not added for its own sake. It comes from exercising the skill that learning ultimately requires. This is why some methods feel productive while producing fragile learning, and others feel frustrating while producing durable learning.

Whether a strategy feels difficult is the wrong question.

The right question is what ability that difficulty is training.

Try This Today

What to do: Choose a topic you studied earlier this week. Instead of reviewing it immediately, wait until some forgetting has occurred. Then try to retrieve the key ideas from memory before opening your notes.

What you may notice: The retrieval attempt will probably feel less fluent than review. You may remember less than expected, and the exercise may feel slower than simply rereading the material.

Why it matters: The effort required to reconstruct information provides information about what is actually accessible. It also gives retrieval another opportunity to strengthen access.

Options Menu

These are the difficulties worth keeping, because each one rehearses an ability the exam will later require. They share the quality Robert and Elizabeth Bjork call desirable difficulty: harder in the moment, stronger over time (Bjork & Bjork, 2011). Pick by what you need to train:

- **Retrieval.** Produce the answer from memory before you check it. Reaching for it is the work the exam asks for, and the reach shows you what is still out of range.

- **Spacing.** Return to material after some forgetting instead of the same evening. The retrieval is harder, and the reconstruction that follows is what strengthens retention (Cepeda et al., 2006).

- **Interleaving.** Mix problem types instead of drilling one topic in a block. Accuracy dips while you work out which problem you are solving, which is the discrimination a vignette later demands (Rohrer & Taylor, 2007).

- **Self-explanation.** Explain a concept aloud, from memory, as if teaching it. The gaps it surfaces are the value (Chi et al., 1994).

- **Productive failure.** Attempt a problem before the instruction arrives. The early struggle builds a framework for the later explanation to attach to (Kapur, 2008).

Common Traps

The difficulty of a session is a poor guide on its own, and a few habits follow from trusting it.

Mistaking suffering for progress assumes that anything hard must be working. Studying on four hours of sleep, or switching constantly between resources, produces difficulty that competes with learning, and that effort goes to waste even when the strain feels like seriousness.

Abandoning a method because it feels worse retreats to whatever feels fluent. The methods that expose gaps tend to be the ones doing the most work, so dropping them the moment they sting throws away the feedback that was about to help.

Adding difficulty for its own sake confuses strain with rigor. A difficulty that does not rehearse a skill you will need later is only more load.

Recap

What to hold onto when a method feels harder than the one before it:

- **Useful difficulty rehearses the skill you will need later.** Difficulty from poor conditions, like lost sleep or constant switching, only drains attention.
- Retrieval, spacing, interleaving, self-explanation, and productive failure feel worse because they ask for more, which is also why they work.
- The question worth asking is what ability a difficulty is training.
- A method that exposes gaps is usually doing its job.
- Forgetting before retrieval is part of the design.

Before You Move On

The previous chapter argued that performance during studying is often a poor measure of learning. This chapter extends that idea by showing that some of the most effective learning strategies can feel less successful while they are happening.

The challenge is introducing the right difficulty in the right place. Making studying as easy as possible was never the target. Some difficulties strengthen learning because they ask students to practice the skills they will eventually need. Others only drain the attention learning depends on.

That observation raises a practical question. If different study strategies train different abilities, how do you decide which strategy fits the task in front of you?

The next chapter turns to that problem by examining how different learning goals require different forms of practice.

References

Bjork, E. L., & Bjork, R. A. (2011). Making things hard on yourself, but in a good way: Creating desirable difficulties to enhance learning. In M. A. Gernsbacher, R. W. Pew, L. M. Hough, & J. R. Pomerantz (Eds.), *Psychology and the real world: Essays illustrating fundamental contributions to society* (pp. 56–64). Worth.

Cepeda, N. J., Pashler, H., Vul, E., Wixted, J. T., & Rohrer, D. (2006). Distributed practice in verbal recall tasks: A review and quantitative synthesis. *Psychological Bulletin, 132*(3), 354–380.

Chi, M. T. H., de Leeuw, N., Chiu, M.-H., & LaVancher, C. (1994). Eliciting self-explanations improves understanding. *Cognitive Science, 18*(3), 439–477.

Dunlosky, J., Rawson, K., Marsh, E., Nathan, M., & Willingham, D. (2013). Improving students' learning with effective learning techniques: Promising directions from cognitive and educational psychology. *Psychological Science in the Public Interest, 14*(1), 4–58.

Kapur, M. (2008). Productive failure. *Cognition and Instruction, 26*(3), 379–424.

Rohrer, D., & Taylor, K. (2007). The shuffling of mathematics problems improves learning. *Instructional Science, 35*(6), 481–498.

CHAPTER SIX

The Best Study Strategy Depends on the Task

Key Question

How do you choose a study method when so many are recommended?

Core Idea

A method works when it matches the specific ability the task is asking you to build.

Example Scenario

Sarah keeps changing study methods. At the beginning of the semester, she commits to flashcards. A few weeks later, she becomes convinced that she should be doing more practice questions. Soon after that, she starts watching additional videos because classmates say they are helpful. By the end of the block, she has tried concept maps, review sheets, question banks, and several different schedules.

Each change is motivated by the same concern: there must be a better way to study. The search is understandable because medical students are surrounded by advice. Classmates recommend resources, upperclassmen share systems, and online forums offer competing opinions about what works best.

For Sarah, the pattern across one block matters more than any single choice. Each switch was a reasonable search for a better tool, made before she had named the learning problem the tool was supposed to solve.

The difficulty is that studying does not work through one universally superior method. The effectiveness of a study strategy depends on what the learner is trying to accomplish. A strategy that works well for memorizing antibiotic coverage may be poorly suited for understanding acid-base physiology, and a strategy that helps distinguish among similar diagnoses may be less useful for building rapid recall.

This chapter argues for a different question. The one to ask is not *What is the best study strategy?* It is *What ability am I trying to build?* That shift moves studying away from the search for a perfect method and toward matching methods to learning goals.

Why Students Search for the Best Method

Students often assume that learning problems are strategy problems. When performance falls short of expectations, the first instinct is frequently to look for a new resource, a new schedule, or a new technique. The assumption is that a better tool will solve the problem.

Sometimes a new strategy helps. A student who relies entirely on review may benefit from retrieval practice, and a student who never uses practice questions may benefit from more application. Research reviews have found that study techniques vary in effectiveness depending on how they are used and what learning outcome they are meant to support (Dunlosky et al., 2013).

The difficulty is that students often change strategies before identifying the learning problem they are trying to solve. As a result, they move from one technique to another without a clear rationale. The process feels productive because action is being taken, but the underlying question remains unanswered.

Before choosing a study method, it helps to understand what kind of learning is required. Different learning goals place different demands on memory, attention, and reasoning. Those demands should guide strategy selection.

Start With the Learning Goal

Students commonly describe their goal as studying a subject. They say they are studying cardiology, pathology, or pharmacology. Those descriptions identify the content, but they do not identify the learning task.

A more practical approach is to ask what the student needs to do with the information. In some situations, the goal is recall. In others, the goal is understanding how concepts fit together. Sometimes the goal is distinguishing among similar possibilities. In clinical settings, the goal may be reasoning through uncertainty.

These distinctions matter because learning activities train different abilities. When students focus only on the content, they risk choosing study methods that do not match the demands of the task. When they focus on the ability being developed, strategy selection becomes more intentional.

The first step is identifying the learning goal clearly enough that the method can be chosen on purpose. Reaching for a resource comes after that.

When the Goal Is Recall

Some medical knowledge must be readily accessible. Drug side effects, diagnostic criteria, microbiology facts, anatomy structures, and laboratory values often fall into this category. Understanding the information is only half of it. The other half is being able to retrieve it when needed.

When recall is the primary goal, retrieval practice is usually one of the most direct approaches available. Practice questions, flashcards, self-testing, and blank-page recall all require students to produce information rather than simply recognize it. Research on retrieval practice suggests that actively retrieving information supports long-term retention, particularly when the material will later need to be retrieved from memory rather than recognized (Roediger & Karpicke, 2006; Karpicke & Blunt, 2011).

This matters because retrieval is itself a skill. Knowledge that cannot be accessed reliably is difficult to use. Students sometimes spend large amounts of time reviewing information that feels familiar while spending relatively little time practicing retrieval.

If the task requires retrieval, then retrieval should be part of the training process. The study method should ask the student to do the same kind of work the exam will later require.

When the Goal Is Understanding

Not every learning task is primarily about memorization. Many topics require students to build explanations and understand relationships among concepts. Heart failure, renal physiology, endocrine regulation, and immunologic mechanisms often require this kind of learning.

Students frequently discover that familiarity is not enough in these situations. They may recognize the information while struggling to explain how the pieces fit together. The gap is rarely lack of exposure. Understanding calls for a different kind of cognitive work.

Activities such as self-explanation, teaching, drawing mechanisms, and explaining concepts in plain language can support this process. These approaches require students to organize knowledge and identify places where understanding remains incomplete, which is part of why explanatory strategies can support deeper learning when used well (Dunlosky et al., 2013).

Knowing the facts is only the start. The aim is understanding how they relate to one another, so the student can use them when the wording, context, or clinical presentation changes.

When the Goal Is Discrimination

Many medical decisions depend on recognizing important differences among similar possibilities. Students must learn to distinguish among diagnoses that share symptoms, medications that appear similar, and disease processes that overlap in important ways.

This type of learning is often more difficult than students expect because familiarity with each option individually does not guarantee the ability to tell them apart. A student may know several diagnoses well and still struggle when they appear together in a question.

Comparative practice can be especially useful in these situations. Instead of studying conditions in isolation, students repeatedly compare alternatives and identify distinguishing features. The learning task shifts from recognition to differentiation.

The important question becomes *Why is this different from the alternatives?* That question helps students move beyond whether a diagnosis looks familiar and toward the reasoning required to choose among plausible options.

When the Goal Is Reasoning

Clinical reasoning requires more than remembering information. Students must gather evidence, interpret findings, evaluate possibilities, and make decisions in situations where uncertainty is unavoidable. Medical education researchers have described expertise as developing through increasingly organized knowledge structures that support efficient reasoning and decision-making (Schmidt & Rikers, 2007).

This type of learning develops gradually. Reading explanations and observing experienced clinicians can be helpful, but reasoning ultimately requires active participation. Students need opportunities to work through cases, justify decisions, and evaluate competing explanations.

Reasoning improves when learners practice reasoning. This is consistent with the broader deliberate-practice literature, which emphasizes that expertise develops through targeted practice, feedback, and repeated work on the specific skills being improved (Ericsson, 2004).

Clinical questions often feel challenging because they require several abilities to work together at the same time. The student may need recall, understanding, discrimination, and judgment inside a single question.

When the Goal Is Building Illness Scripts

Many students assume that expertise develops primarily through accumulating more facts. Experts certainly know more than novices, but expertise also involves organizing knowledge differently.

Medical education researchers describe this process through the development of illness scripts (Schmidt & Rikers, 2007; Charlin et al., 2007). An illness script is a structured mental representation of a disease. It includes typical symptoms, risk factors, physical findings, disease mechanisms, and common clinical patterns.

A novice studying heart failure may remember dozens of disconnected facts. An experienced clinician often sees a pattern. Shortness of breath, orthopnea, lower-extremity edema, elevated jugular venous pressure, and reduced exercise tolerance become part of a coherent clinical story.

This helps explain why clinical questions feel different from basic science questions. The work is no longer retrieving facts. It is recognizing which pattern best fits the information available.

As training progresses, students become less dependent on isolated facts and increasingly rely on these organized knowledge structures. Learning organizes facts into usable patterns.

Next action: when studying a disease, ask what findings belong together instead of memorizing each finding separately.

Choosing Methods More Intentionally

No single tool is best, because each has both strengths and limits. Flashcards train recall efficiently but may not build a full explanatory model unless used that way. Practice questions support reasoning, and they often expose gaps that send the student back to explanation. Once the learning goal is clear, the choice follows from it. Studying becomes a design decision: choose the method that trains the ability the task requires.

Try This Today

What to do: Before beginning your next study session, write down the primary ability you are trying to develop. Decide whether the goal is recall, understanding, discrimination, or reasoning. Then choose a study activity that directly trains that ability.

What you may notice: The study method you usually use may not be the method that best fits the task. Different learning goals often require different forms of practice, and a familiar method may feel comfortable even when it is poorly matched to the work in front of you.

Why it matters: Effective studying depends less on finding the best strategy and more on selecting a strategy that matches the demands of the task. The method should train the ability you will eventually need to perform.

Options Menu

The point of the chapter is that the method should match the ability. These are concrete ways to do that, each a reading or study technique aimed at one goal and adapted for closed-book, vignette-style exams. Matching the reading approach to the purpose in this way is the core of flexible reading (McWhorter & Sember, 2020). Pick by the ability the task demands:

- **For recall: read to retrieve.** Preview a section, close it, and produce the facts from memory before checking. The reading ends in retrieval, which is the work the exam rewards (Roediger & Karpicke, 2006).
- **For understanding: survey, question, recite.** Turn a mechanism chapter's headings into questions before reading, then recite the answers from memory and review what you missed. The sequence is Robinson's SQ3R method (Robinson, 1946).
- **For discrimination: read comparatively.** Study two look-alikes side by side and build a chart of the findings that separate them. The task moves toward the differentiation a *which diagnosis* question requires.
- **For reasoning: work the case first.** Attempt the question, commit to an answer, then read to find where the reasoning broke.

Working a problem before the explanation builds reasoning a read-through alone does not (Ericsson, 2004).

- **For illness scripts: read for the pattern.** As you study a disease, group the findings that travel together into a clinical story rather than memorizing them separately (Schmidt & Rikers, 2007).

Common Traps

The search for a better method is reasonable, and a few versions of it quietly backfire.

Switching methods before naming the learning problem chases the hope that a better tool will fix things. Changing the technique without identifying what kind of learning is failing leaves the next method matched no better than the last, and the motion feels like progress while the question stays open.

Using one method for every goal holds onto the comfort of a familiar tool. Flashcards for a reasoning task, or rereading for a recall task, trains the wrong ability efficiently. What fails is the match to the task, and no amount of effort fixes a mismatch.

Choosing by popularity outsources the decision to classmates. A resource that suits someone else's current gap may not suit yours, because the right method depends on the ability you need to build.

Recap

What to hold onto when you are tempted to change methods again:

- **There is no single best study method**, because there is no single learning task.

- **Name the ability first (recall**, understanding, discrimination, reasoning), then choose the method that trains it.

- The method should ask for the same work the exam will: production for recall, explanation for understanding, comparison for discrimination, case-work for reasoning.

- Switching methods before naming the problem feels productive and rarely is.

- **Expertise grows through organization as much as accumulation**, so study the pattern, not only the facts.

Before You Move On

This chapter has focused on matching learning strategies to the abilities students are trying to develop.

The central idea is simple. There is no universally best study method because there is no universally identical learning task. Different goals require different forms of practice.

This observation creates another challenge. Even when students choose appropriate strategies, they still need to determine whether their judgments about learning are accurate. The next chapter examines calibration and explores why confidence and competence do not always move together.

References

Charlin, B., Boshuizen, H. P. A., Custers, E. J., & Feltovich, P. J. (2007). Scripts and clinical reasoning. *Medical Education, 41*(12), 1178–1184.

Dunlosky, J., Rawson, K., Marsh, E., Nathan, M., & Willingham, D. (2013). Improving students' learning with effective learning techniques: Promising directions from cognitive and educational psychology. *Psychological Science in the Public Interest, 14*(1), 4–58.

Ericsson, K. A. (2004). Deliberate practice and the acquisition and maintenance of expert performance in medicine and related domains. *Academic Medicine, 79*(10 Suppl), S70–S81.

Karpicke, J. D., & Blunt, J. R. (2011). Retrieval practice produces more learning than elaborative studying with concept mapping. *Science, 331*(6018), 772–775.

McWhorter, K. T., & Sember, B. M. (2020). *College reading and study skills* (14th ed.). Pearson.

Robinson, F. P. (1946). *Effective study.* Harper & Brothers.

Roediger, H. L., III, & Karpicke, J. D. (2006). Test-enhanced learning: Taking memory tests improves long-term retention. *Psychological Science, 17*(3), 249–255.

Schmidt, H. G., & Rikers, R. M. J. P. (2007). How expertise develops in medicine: Knowledge encapsulation and illness script formation. *Medical Education, 41*(12), 1133–1139.

CHAPTER SEVEN

Knowing It Is Not the Same as Using It

Key Question

Why can you know the material and still miss the diagnosis when the patient does not look like the question?

Core Idea

Knowledge does not automatically travel to new situations. Transfer is a separate skill, and it is shaped by how you practice, not simply by how much you know.

Example Scenario

Tomas scored in the top quartile on the cardiology block. He can draw the pressure-volume loop from memory and recite the compensatory mechanisms in heart failure without hesitation.

On his first medicine rotation, an eighty-year-old woman is admitted with fatigue, poor appetite, and mild confusion. She mentions that she has been sleeping on two pillows. The attending asks Tomas what he thinks is going on, and nothing arrives.

Afterward, reading the note, he sees it at once. Orthopnea. Volume overload. The presentation he could have explained in detail three weeks ago, wearing clothes he had never seen it wear.

Tomas draws the conclusion the moment invites: *I must not have learned it as well as I thought.*

The knowledge held. What had never been practiced was the walk from a tired woman on two pillows back to the diagram he knew by heart.

The Gap Between the Desk and the Ward

A student can master a block, perform well on its exams, and then stall in front of a real patient presenting the same disease in an unfamiliar way. The knowledge is there. It simply does not arrive when the situation looks different from where it was learned.

This is the problem of *transfer*: applying what you learned in one context to a new one. It is different from the access problem described earlier. Access is about reaching stored knowledge under pressure. Transfer is about recognizing when that knowledge applies after the surface details have changed and the cues you rehearsed are no longer present.

The distinction matters because medical training is fundamentally a transfer task. The exam vignette, the patient on the ward, and the future clinic visit will never look exactly like the paragraph you studied. Learning that remains tied to its original wording has limited value in a profession where the wording is always changing.

Why Transfer Is Harder Than It Looks

Researchers distinguish between *near transfer*, in which a new situation closely resembles the original, and *far transfer*, in which it does not (Barnett & Ceci, 2002). Near transfer is common. Far transfer is considerably more difficult.

That finding is worth stating plainly. Decades of research suggest that knowledge does not automatically generalize to new contexts, even when it has been learned well. A student may accurately explain a mechanism in the abstract yet fail to recognize it in a patient who has never looked like the textbook example.

One reason is that learning naturally becomes attached to the context in which it was acquired. A concept studied only through cardiology questions can become quietly linked to cardiology-shaped cues. When the same mechanism appears in a different clinical context, it may not immediately be recognized as the same underlying idea.

This does not mean transfer is impossible. It means transfer usually has to be built into practice instead of being left to emerge on its own.

What Improves Transfer?

Several study habits consistently improve the likelihood that knowledge will transfer. Each changes the way you practice, and none of them depends on adding hours.

The first is comparing contrasting cases. When two cases share similar surface features but differ in their underlying mechanisms, studying them side by side encourages learners to identify the principle that separates them. Studying those same cases independently is much less likely to produce that abstraction (Gick & Holyoak, 1983). Comparing dyspnea caused by heart failure with dyspnea caused by COPD, for example, trains the discrimination that real patients require.

The second is studying in the direction of use. In practice, patients present with symptoms, and the diagnosis is what you are there to work out. Practicing from presentation to diagnosis (*Here is the patient. What is happening?*) rehearses the retrieval pathway you will actually use. Studying only from disease to features rehearses a pathway you will use far less often (Schwartz & Bransford, 1998).

The third is variability of practice. Encountering the same mechanism across several different patient presentations gradually loosens it from any single example. Over time, the knowledge becomes available as a general principle instead of the memory of one familiar vignette. Practice feels less tidy, but the knowledge becomes more flexible.

When the Bedside Feels Harder Than the Desk

Transfer fits naturally into the developmental picture described earlier. As expertise develops, biomedical knowledge becomes encapsulated into illness scripts and, eventually, into rapid pattern recognition (Schmidt & Rikers, 2007). Each step represents knowledge becoming usable farther from the context in which it was first learned.

It also sets a realistic expectation. Because far transfer is inherently difficult, a student who performs smoothly at the desk but hesitates at the bedside is not necessarily showing a knowledge deficit. More often, they are encountering the ordinary challenge of applying knowledge across contexts. The response is usually to practice that transition. Relearning the material rarely addresses it.

Try This Today

What to do: Choose one concept you studied this week. Find two cases that appear similar on the surface but differ in their underlying mechanisms. Before checking any resource, write one sentence explaining the difference.

What you may notice: The distinction is often harder to describe than the definition itself. That difficulty is the point. It reflects the discrimination real clinical reasoning requires.

Why it matters: Comparing contrasting cases strengthens the abstraction that transfer depends on. Studying them separately rarely has the same effect.

Options Menu

Transfer is built during practice. Nothing gets added afterward. Reach for whichever fits:

- **Compare, do not just collect.** Study similar-looking cases side by side and name the underlying difference. It is slower than reviewing them in turn, and the comparison is what generalizes. Exposure alone does not (Gick & Holyoak, 1983).

- **Study in the direction of use.** Practice moving from presentation to diagnosis, and not only from disease to features. It feels less orderly, and it mirrors the path a patient actually presents.

• **Vary the context.** Encounter the same mechanism in several different patient stories. The extra examples cost time, and they loosen the principle from any single vignette so it travels.

• **State the rule without the case.** After a worked example, write the general principle independent of that patient's details. It is an extra step, and it is where the transferable part lives.

Common Traps

Several reasonable study habits can quietly keep knowledge tied to where it was learned.

Treating fluency on question banks as readiness for patients assumes the two are the same task. Question banks often measure near transfer, while clinical work frequently demands something farther.

Studying each topic in a single, orderly block feels efficient, but it also strengthens the cues unique to that block. The same organization that makes studying feel smooth can make later application more difficult.

After struggling with a patient, it is tempting to relearn the content from the beginning. Sometimes that is appropriate. Often, however, the knowledge itself is intact, and what needs practice is applying it across different contexts.

Recap

What to remember when you know the material on paper but struggle to use it in the room:

• Transfer is a separate skill from storing or accessing knowledge.

• **Far transfer is genuinely difficult**, so a gap between desk performance and bedside performance is expected, and it diagnoses nothing about the learner.

• Comparing contrasting cases strengthens the discrimination real patients require.

• Practicing toward use and across varied contexts gives knowledge a better chance of traveling.

Before You Move On

The previous chapter matched study methods to learning goals. This chapter asked a different question: what happens after learning succeeds?

Knowledge does not automatically travel from one setting to another. Transfer develops through comparison, varied practice, and rehearsal in the direction the knowledge will eventually be used. Even then, it remains imperfect.

That has an important consequence. If knowledge arrives unevenly across situations, confidence becomes an unreliable guide to what you can actually do. The next chapter explores that problem directly, examining why the feeling of knowing is often a poor measure of whether knowledge will be available when you need it most.

References

Barnett, S. M., & Ceci, S. J. (2002). When and where do we apply what we learn? A taxonomy for far transfer. *Psychological Bulletin, 128*(4), 612–637.

Gick, M. L., & Holyoak, K. J. (1983). Schema induction and analogical transfer. *Cognitive Psychology, 15*(1), 1–38.

Schmidt, H. G., & Rikers, R. M. J. P. (2007). How expertise develops in medicine: Knowledge encapsulation and illness script formation. *Medical Education, 41*(12), 1133–1139.

Schwartz, D. L., & Bransford, J. D. (1998). A time for telling. *Cognition and Instruction, 16*(4), 475–522.

CHAPTER EIGHT

Confidence Is Information, Not Proof

Key Question

How much should confidence guide what you study next?

Core Idea

Confidence is a signal worth testing, because the feeling of knowing and the ability to retrieve can come apart.

Example Scenario

Priya finishes a long study session feeling encouraged.

She reviewed her notes, recognized most of the material, and moved through the chapter more quickly than she expected. By the end of the evening, she feels confident that the information is well learned. The familiarity is reassuring because it creates a sense of progress.

A few days later, she sits down to complete practice questions. The experience is unexpectedly frustrating. Concepts that felt clear during review suddenly seem difficult to retrieve. Details that appeared familiar are harder to access than she anticipated.

Plenty of students recognize Priya's two evenings. What they expose is the distance this chapter is about: the confidence she left with and the access she actually had were two different readings of the same material.

Why Confidence Feels Reliable

Confidence plays an important role in learning.

Students constantly make judgments about what they understand, what they remember, and what still requires attention. Without those judgments, studying would become inefficient because every topic would appear equally important.

The difficulty is that confidence is an internal experience, and no internal experience directly measures learning (Eva & Regehr, 2005). Students do not observe memory itself. They observe feelings associated with memory. Those feelings can be useful, but they are not always accurate.

One reason confidence feels persuasive is that familiarity often feels similar to mastery. Material that has been reviewed repeatedly becomes easier to recognize. Processing feels smoother. Concepts seem clearer. The experience creates the impression that learning has occurred.

Sometimes that impression is correct. Sometimes familiarity reflects exposure more than accessibility.

The challenge is learning how to distinguish between the two.

The Difference Between Recognition and Retrieval

Recognition and retrieval feel similar from the inside but are different processes: information can feel familiar when it is shown to you and still be impossible to produce without cues. Because recognition is the easier of the two, it can create false confidence, and the gap appears the moment a question offers nothing to recognize. Research on retrieval practice has repeatedly shown that recognizing information is not the same as retrieving it independently (Roediger & Karpicke, 2006; Karpicke & Blunt, 2011), and most examinations require the second.

Why Familiarity Feels Like Learning

Students often judge learning by how easy studying feels, yet ease during study and success during retrieval are not the same outcome. Robert and Elizabeth Bjork have argued that conditions producing strong feelings of fluency do not always produce durable learning (Bjork & Bjork, 2011). Fluency during review is real, and it is best read as one signal among several. It proves nothing about what will still be accessible later.

Why Low Confidence Can Also Be Misleading

Students often assume that inaccurate judgments only occur when confidence is too high.

The opposite problem is also common.

Some students underestimate what they know. They complete practice questions successfully while remaining convinced that they are unprepared. They interpret uncertainty as evidence that learning is incomplete.

This tendency is especially common in environments where standards are high and knowledge is always expanding. Medical students are continuously exposed to information they do not yet know. As a result, they may focus more on gaps than on what has already been learned.

Low confidence sometimes reflects genuine uncertainty. In other cases, it reflects awareness of complexity instead of absence of knowledge.

The feeling alone cannot determine which explanation is correct.

Why Calibration Matters

Chapter Four introduced calibration as the check on how well your sense of knowing matches what you can actually do. This chapter takes up what happens when the two disagree.

Well-calibrated students estimate what they know and what they do not know with reasonable accuracy. Certainty is never the standard. Their judgments allow them to allocate attention efficiently because they can identify weaknesses without overlooking strengths.

Poor calibration creates problems in both directions.

Overconfidence can lead students to stop studying material that still requires work. Underconfidence can lead students to spend excessive time reviewing information they already understand. In both cases, study time becomes less efficient.

Educational researchers have found that metacognitive monitoring plays an important role in self-regulated learning because decisions about studying depend partly on judgments about learning (Dunlosky & Metcalfe, 2009).

Accurate calibration supports better decisions.

Testing Creates Better Information

Students often rely on feelings when evaluating learning because feelings are immediately available.

Feelings provide indirect evidence. Retrieval provides direct evidence. Practice questions, self-testing, teaching, and free recall all create opportunities to observe performance instead of estimating it. These activities make strengths and weaknesses more visible.

Testing serves two functions at the same time. It strengthens learning through retrieval practice, and it improves calibration by providing feedback about what is actually accessible (Roediger & Karpicke, 2006).

This is one reason practice questions are so valuable. They reveal information that familiarity alone cannot provide.

Students may not always enjoy what the results show, but the information is often useful.

Using Confidence Wisely

Confidence is worth listening to.

Eliminating confidence, or replacing it with constant skepticism, would cost you a useful signal. Confidence provides information about how learning feels. That information has value.

The challenge is remembering that confidence is one source of information, and never the final authority. Feelings become more useful when combined with evidence from retrieval, application, and performance.

Students often improve calibration by asking whether confidence is supported by observable performance. A feeling of preparedness becomes more informative when it is accompanied by successful retrieval. A feeling of uncertainty becomes easier to interpret when it is compared with actual results.

Perfect self-assessment is out of reach.

The objective is judgments accurate enough to guide learning.

Confidence Problems and Identity Problems Are Not the Same Thing

Medical students often assume that feelings of inadequacy reflect deficiencies in knowledge. Sometimes they do. Sometimes the problem is different.

Psychologist E. Tory Higgins proposed Self-Discrepancy Theory to explain how distress emerges when people compare who they are with who they believe they should be (Higgins, 1987).

Medical students often manage three versions of themselves simultaneously. The first is the actual self: where they are now. The second is the ideal self: the physician they hope to become. The third is the ought self: the student they believe they should already be.

Much of the emotional strain in medical training occurs in the distance between these versions.

A student may correctly answer most questions while feeling inadequate because the comparison target is perfection instead of progress. Another may interpret normal uncertainty as evidence of failure because they believe competent students should not feel uncertain.

Some of these experiences are discrepancy problems wearing the clothes of a confidence problem.

Reducing unnecessary self-judgment leaves the standards where they are. What changes is the accuracy of the picture you hold of your own development.

Next action: when self-criticism appears, ask whether it reflects current performance or comparison with an unrealistic standard.

Try This Today

What to do: Before completing a question block, practice quiz, or retrieval exercise, estimate how many questions you expect to answer correctly. Write down the prediction before beginning.

After finishing, compare the prediction with the actual result.

What you may notice: Confidence and performance often differ more than expected. Some topics may feel stronger than they are, while others may be more secure than they feel.

Why it matters: Calibration improves when students repeatedly compare predictions with outcomes. The process creates feedback that helps confidence become more accurate over time.

Options Menu

The shift turns one feeling into evidence, and these are other ways to keep confidence honest. Each surfaces the distance between how learning feels and what is actually accessible. If helpful:

- **Tag your confidence before you check.** On a question block, mark how sure you were on each item, then look at which *sure* answers were wrong. The extra step shows precisely where confidence misleads you.

- **Test the topics that feel safe.** Quiz the material you would otherwise skip because it feels solid. Overconfidence tends to hide in exactly the topics you would not revisit.

- **Explain, then verify.** Explain a concept from memory, then check your notes for what came out vague or wrong. Explaining separates feeling clear from being right.

- **Compare confidence with a result.** When a topic feels shaky, run a few questions before treating the unease as proof you do not know it. Testing turns the feeling into something you can check (Roediger & Karpicke, 2006).

Common Traps

Confidence is a useful signal, and the traps come from treating it as more than a signal.

Taking high confidence as proof of learning lets you stop studying what feels done. Familiarity feels almost identical to mastery from the inside, so the topics that feel most finished are often the ones still quietly fragile.

Taking low confidence as proof you do not know something sends you back over material you already hold. In a field where you are always surrounded by what you have not yet learned, that unease often reflects awareness of complexity rather than absence of knowledge.

Measuring yourself against the student you think you should already be turns ordinary progress into evidence of inadequacy. That is a discrepancy between selves more than a gap in knowledge, and it answers to a different response.

Recap

What to hold onto when confidence and results disagree:

- **Confidence reports how learning feels**, which is useful information, and it never measures what has been learned.
- **Recognition and retrieval feel alike from the inside**, and most exams require the second.
- Calibration can fail in both directions: overconfidence stops needed work, underconfidence wastes time on what is already known.
- **Testing converts a feeling into evidence**, so predict, then check.
- **Feeling behind and being behind can come apart**, so compare the feeling with an actual result.

Before You Move On

This chapter examined calibration and the relationship between confidence and performance.

Confidence is useful because it helps students make decisions about learning. The challenge is that confidence reflects perception, and perception is not observation. Familiarity, fluency, and uncertainty can all influence judgments in ways that are not fully aligned with actual performance.

Learning becomes easier to evaluate when students combine confidence with evidence. Retrieval, testing, and feedback provide information that feelings alone cannot supply.

Understanding learning is only part of the challenge. Students must also understand how they interpret their experiences while learning. The next chapter begins that transition by examining why academic struggles so often become personal judgments about ability, worth, and belonging.

References

Bjork, E. L., & Bjork, R. A. (2011). Making things hard on yourself, but in a good way: Creating desirable difficulties to enhance learning. In M. A. Gernsbacher, R. W. Pew, L. M. Hough, & J. R. Pomerantz (Eds.), *Psychology and the real world: Essays illustrating fundamental contributions to society* (pp. 56–64). Worth.

Dunlosky, J., & Metcalfe, J. (2009). *Metacognition.* Sage.

Eva, K. W., & Regehr, G. (2005). Self-assessment in the health professions: A reformulation and research agenda. *Academic Medicine, 80*(10 Suppl), S46–S54.

Higgins, E. T. (1987). Self-discrepancy: A theory relating self and affect. *Psychological Review, 94*(3), 319–340.

Karpicke, J. D., & Blunt, J. R. (2011). Retrieval practice produces more learning than elaborative studying with concept mapping. *Science, 331*(6018), 772–775.

Roediger, H. L., III, & Karpicke, J. D. (2006). Test-enhanced learning: Taking memory tests improves long-term retention. *Psychological Science, 17*(3), 249–255.

CHAPTER NINE

Why Smart Medical Students Misread Their Own Experience

Key Question

Why do capable students misjudge how well their studying is working?

Core Idea

Several common study experiences feel like learning while building little access.

Example Scenario

Wei spends an evening on the nephrotic syndromes. By the end, minimal change disease, focal segmental glomerulosclerosis, membranous nephropathy, and diabetic nephropathy all feel comfortably familiar, and he closes his notes feeling prepared. The next morning a question presents a patient without naming the diagnosis, the answer choices look unfamiliar, and the distinctions that felt obvious the night before will not come.

What happens to Wei plays out the whole chapter in a single night. The reassurance he felt was real, and it came from familiarity instead of the access a question requires.

Five Familiar Misreadings

Most of the ways students misjudge their own learning are versions of the same move, and the earlier chapters have already named them. Research on self-regulated learning has catalogued these illusions and their persistence (Bjork et al., 2013). They are worth gathering in one place, briefly, before turning to two that this chapter takes up in full.

The fluency illusion treats recognition as mastery. Material that has been reviewed often feels smooth, and that smoothness reads as knowing, until a question asks for production rather than recognition. Chapter Three is the fuller account.

The effort illusion treats difficulty as failure. When retrieval feels slow and uneven, students conclude the method is not working, when often it is simply exposing weaknesses that review had kept hidden. Chapter Five describes why that difficulty is frequently the useful kind.

The confidence illusion treats certainty as accuracy. A lecture that made sense while it was being explained can feel like settled knowledge, even though the feeling of knowing and the ability to retrieve are only loosely related. Chapter Eight examines this directly.

Single-question overgeneralization turns one vivid moment into a global verdict. A question missed on rounds becomes evidence about an entire field. Clinical-reasoning research has shown repeatedly that performance is highly case-specific, so a single result predicts far less than it seems to (Norman, 2005; Norman et al., 2006). Chapter Three's point that a question is a sample applies here as well.

Social comparison turns other students into the measuring stick. Their visible confidence becomes evidence that everyone else is further along, even though almost everything that produced it stays out of view. Chapter Thirteen takes up comparison in full.

Each of these is the same underlying pattern: a feeling, quietly promoted to evidence. The two that follow are worth examining more closely, because they shape clinical learning in particular.

Outcome Bias

When Results Rewrite the Story

Medical training generates a constant stream of outcomes. Questions are answered correctly or incorrectly. Presentations receive praise or criticism. Shelf scores rise and fall. Because outcomes are highly visible, students naturally use them to evaluate their learning.

The difficulty is that outcomes do not reveal how those outcomes were produced.

Kahneman (2011) describes outcome bias as the tendency to judge decisions through their results, with little attention to the quality of the reasoning that generated them. This tendency creates problems in education because correct answers and good reasoning are not identical.

A student may answer a difficult infectious disease question correctly after recognizing a familiar phrase in the stem. Another student may construct a thoughtful differential diagnosis and miss the question because of one forgotten detail.

If both learners focus only on the outcome, both may learn the wrong lesson. The first may become overly confident in weak reasoning. The second may lose trust in a process that was largely sound.

Assessment does more than determine whether an answer was correct. It offers a chance to understand how that answer emerged. Students who review only outcomes often miss the most valuable information available to them.

Strong learners become curious about process. They ask whether success resulted from reasoning, recognition, pattern matching, or guessing. They examine whether an error reflected a conceptual misunderstanding, a factual gap, or a momentary lapse. These questions are often more informative than the score itself.

Outcomes matter because they provide feedback. Yet learning accelerates when students become interested in the reasoning that produced those outcomes.

The Clinical Exposure Illusion

When Seeing a Case Feels Like Learning a Case

Perhaps the most important illusion in clinical education is the belief that exposure automatically produces expertise.

The assumption sounds reasonable because medicine is learned through patients. Students spend years moving through hospitals, clinics, and wards. Every encounter appears to add another piece to the puzzle.

Exposure is unquestionably important. Without exposure, expertise cannot develop. The mistake occurs when exposure is confused with learning itself.

A student may spend an afternoon caring for a patient with decompensated heart failure. The symptoms are memorable, the teaching is excellent, and the experience feels meaningful. By the end of the shift, the student may feel that heart failure is now understood.

Several weeks later, a different patient presents with overlapping symptoms. The diagnosis is less obvious, and the familiar pattern does not immediately appear. The student discovers that remembering a case and understanding a condition are different achievements.

According to Schmidt and Rikers (2007), expertise develops through the gradual formation of illness scripts that organize clinical knowledge into patterns that can be recognized and applied across different contexts. Charlin and colleagues (2007) similarly emphasize that clinical reasoning depends on structured knowledge, which isolated encounters do not supply.

Exposure provides the raw material. Reflection organizes it, comparison sharpens it, and retrieval stabilizes it. Over time, those processes turn individual encounters into clinical expertise. Students often assume that seeing a diagnosis is enough, when meaningful learning usually occurs after the encounter, as the learner compares cases, identifies distinguishing features, reconstructs reasoning, and integrates new information into existing knowledge.

The patient encounter begins the process. Completing it is separate work.

Bringing It Together

The feelings themselves carry useful information. The difficulty comes when they become the final judge of learning. Strong learners hold their experiences more loosely, staying curious about what a feeling might mean before accepting the first interpretation.

That habit sounds modest, and it grows more important as training progresses. Clinical expertise depends on acquiring knowledge and on judging accurately what has and has not been learned. Learning and the feeling of learning are different things, and much of professional development is becoming better at telling them apart.

It is worth being honest about what the training environment rewards. The visible signals get the reinforcement: a quick answer on rounds, a confident manner, hours logged. Those are exactly the signals this chapter shows to be unreliable. What actually predicts competence is evidence gathered over time, which is mostly invisible in the moment. Trusting the visible signal is a reasonable response to an environment that displays it so prominently. Noticing the gap is what lets you give weight to the quieter, better evidence.

Try This Today

What to do: Take one strong impression from today's studying or clinical work (*this is solid*, *I am behind*, *that session was wasted*) and before acting on it, name one piece of evidence for or against it. A cold retrieval attempt, a recent score, or a comparison with last month will do.

What you may notice: The feeling and the evidence often disagree, and the feeling tends to be more certain than the evidence supports.

Why it matters: Every misreading in this chapter is a feeling treated as proof. Asking for the evidence is the single habit that interrupts all of them.

Options Menu

Every misreading in this chapter is a feeling promoted to evidence, so one move answers all of them: ask what the evidence shows before you act. Keep a few questions ready for the moment a feeling arrives dressed as a fact.

- **That felt familiar.** *Can I produce it without looking?* Catches the fluency illusion, before a smooth evening becomes a surprising morning.

- **I feel sure about this.** *What is my evidence?* Catches the confidence illusion, where certainty and accuracy come apart.

- **That block felt awful.** *What did it actually show me?* Catches the effort illusion, where the difficulty that exposes gaps gets read as failure.

- **One question went badly.** *What can one question actually tell me?* Catches single-question overgeneralization. Performance is case-specific.

- **They seem further along.** *What am I actually comparing?* Catches social comparison, where visible confidence hides everything that produced it.

Common Traps

The misreadings in this chapter share a few practical forms.

Treating a smooth session as proof of learning lets familiarity stand in for access, which is why a confident evening so often precedes a surprising morning.

Reading difficulty as failure retreats from the very methods that were working, because the strategies that expose gaps are usually the ones doing the most.

Drawing a global conclusion from one vivid moment closes the question early. Performance is case-specific, and a single case rarely carries the meaning a strong feeling assigns it.

Recap

What to hold onto when a feeling arrives looking like a fact:

- Learning is invisible, so the signals you read instead (familiarity, effort, confidence, a single result) are clues, and none of them is a measurement.
- Each misreading is the same move: a feeling treated as evidence.
- **The habit that helps is asking**, before acting, what the evidence shows.
- **Outcomes tell you what happened**, and the reasoning behind a result is where the learning is.
- Seeing a case begins the work of learning it.

Before You Move On

This chapter gathered the ways studying can feel like learning while building little access. Each one is the same move, a feeling promoted to evidence, and each answers to the same correction: ask what the evidence shows before acting on the impression.

Reading your own experience accurately is harder than it sounds, because the feelings involved carry weight. A missed question stings. A smooth session reassures. A classmate's confidence lands somewhere personal.

The next part of the book takes those feelings seriously. Anxiety, self-doubt, and avoidance sit inside the learning system, drawing on the same capacity that studying requires and shaping what a student can do with it.

References

Bjork, R. A., Dunlosky, J., & Kornell, N. (2013). Self-regulated learning: Beliefs, techniques, and illusions. *Annual Review of Psychology, 64*, 417–444.

Charlin, B., Boshuizen, H. P. A., Custers, E. J., & Feltovich, P. J. (2007). Scripts and clinical reasoning. *Medical Education, 41*(12), 1178–1184.

Kahneman, D. (2011). *Thinking, fast and slow*. Farrar, Straus and Giroux.

Norman, G. (2005). Research in clinical reasoning: Past history and current trends. *Medical Education, 39*(4), 418–427.

Norman, G., Bordage, G., Page, G., & Keane, D. (2006). How specific is case specificity? *Medical Education, 40*(7), 618–623.

Schmidt, H. G., & Rikers, R. M. J. P. (2007). How expertise develops in medicine: Knowledge encapsulation and illness script formation. *Medical Education, 41*(12), 1133–1139.

PART THREE

Emotion Is Not Noise

Part Two focused on study design: reducing load, training retrieval, matching strategies to tasks, and reading performance data more accurately. These changes matter. They also do not remove the conditions in which medical students actually study.

Learning happens with anxiety in the room. It happens after disappointing scores, during comparison, after long days, and in the presence of shame, avoidance, fatigue, and pressure. These experiences are not separate from studying. They shape what attention can hold, what memory can access, and whether a session begins at all.

Emotion changes what attention can hold, what memory can retrieve, and what a student is able to attempt. It is not separate from learning. It is one of the conditions learning happens inside. If cognitive load limits what working memory can manage, emotional threat can consume some of that same capacity, and a study plan can be technically sound and still fail when there is not enough mental room left to use it.

Part Three begins with a problem many students recognize immediately: the experience of knowing something and then being unable to reach it when it matters. Chapter Ten examines why students blank during questions, exams, presentations, and other high-pressure moments. Chapter Eleven then turns to anxiety, not as a separate issue from learning, but as a condition that can change attention, memory, and performance. Together, these chapters explore how pressure influences access to knowledge and how students often misinterpret the resulting difficulties.

CHAPTER TEN

Why You Blank When It Matters Most

Key Question

Why does knowledge you clearly have disappear under pressure?

Core Idea

Pressure consumes the working memory retrieval depends on, so well-learned material can briefly become unreachable.

Example Scenario

On rounds, the attending turns to Omar with a question he has reviewed a dozen times. For a moment, nothing comes. The blank feels total, and a quick conclusion follows: *I never really knew this.*

The blank Omar hits says less about what he learned than about the moment he is in. Pressure itself taxes the working memory retrieval depends on: the knowledge did not disappear, the room to reach it narrowed.

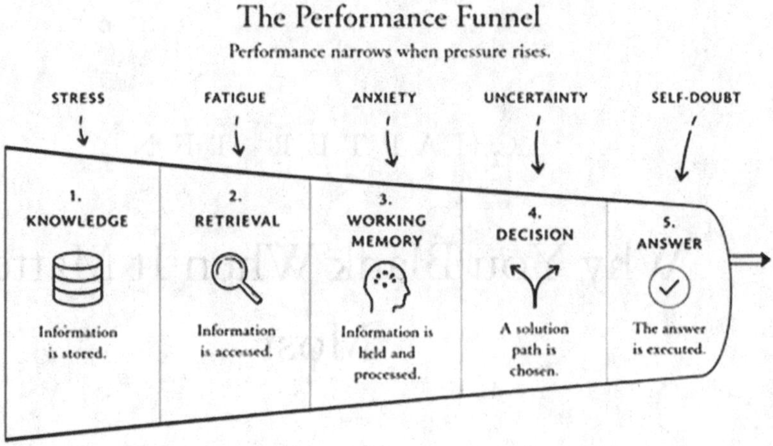

Figure 5. The conditions surrounding retrieval influence whether stored knowledge can be used.

The Hidden Cost of Pressure

Figure 5 illustrates how pressure can affect performance at every stage between stored knowledge and producing an answer. When stakes are low, attention is often directed outward toward the task. A student reads a question, analyzes the information, and searches memory for relevant knowledge. Most available cognitive resources can be devoted to reasoning and retrieval.

High-pressure situations often change that balance.

As the perceived importance of the task increases, attention frequently shifts inward. Students begin monitoring their own performance. They wonder whether they are doing well enough. They think about the consequences of failure. They notice physical symptoms of anxiety and begin evaluating what those symptoms might mean.

These thoughts feel automatic because, in many ways, they are.

Self-monitoring, though, requires mental resources. Working memory, the limited system that supports active thinking and reasoning, must now manage both the task and the student's reaction to the task. Beilock and Carr (2005) demonstrated that pressure can impair performance by consuming working-memory resources that would otherwise support problem solving and retrieval.

The result is a cognitive traffic jam. The knowledge may still be present, but access becomes less reliable because attention is being pulled in multiple directions at once.

When Knowing and Accessing Become Different Problems

Students often assume that memory is either present or absent. If they cannot retrieve something during an examination, they conclude that the knowledge does not exist.

Human memory is rarely that simple.

Many students have experienced the peculiar frustration of remembering an answer immediately after an examination ends. The forgotten fact appears during the walk to the parking lot, while discussing questions with classmates, or even while opening the door to leave the testing center.

These moments are often interpreted as evidence that the brain is somehow unfair or unpredictable.

The likelier interpretation is that retrieval conditions changed. Once the examination ended, the pressure associated with performance diminished. Attention no longer needed to monitor consequences, evaluate performance, or anticipate outcomes. Cognitive resources that had been occupied by stress-related thoughts became available again.

The information was likely present all along. What changed was that the pathway to it became easier to reach.

This distinction matters because students frequently underestimate how much retrieval depends on context. The inability to access knowledge under pressure does not automatically prove that learning failed to occur.

Why Anxiety Feels So Convincing

Anxiety is persuasive because it feels diagnostic. When students feel anxious before an examination, they often assume the emotion is revealing something important about their preparation.

Sometimes it is.

More often, anxiety reflects the significance of the task rather than the quality of preparation.

A student can study thoroughly, complete practice questions successfully, and still feel anxious before a high-stakes examination. The emotional response emerges because the outcome matters. Medical students care about performance, future opportunities, evaluations, and professional identity. It would be surprising if important events produced no emotional response at all.

The difficulty arises when anxiety is interpreted as evidence. A student notices nervousness and immediately concludes that preparation must be inadequate. That conclusion creates additional worry, which consumes additional working-memory resources, which increases the likelihood of retrieval difficulties. The cycle becomes self-reinforcing.

The original anxiety is no longer the problem. The meaning attached to it becomes the problem.

The Monitoring Trap

Under normal conditions, many cognitive skills run efficiently and largely automatically. Students read vignettes, recognize patterns, and retrieve information without consciously supervising each step. Pressure encourages interference with that process. Baumeister's early work on choking traced this to self-focus: pressure pulls conscious attention onto the performer's own execution, which can disrupt processes that normally run smoothly on their own (Baumeister, 1984). Attention shifts from solving the problem toward evaluating the person solving it, and resources spent on self-evaluation are no longer available for reasoning and retrieval.

Why Practice Sometimes Fails to Predict Performance

When practice performance and examination performance do not match, students often assume the gap reflects poor preparation. The explanation is sometimes simpler. Practice and testing place different demands on cognition: at home a student can devote nearly all attention to reasoning, while a high-stakes examination redirects some of it toward worry and performance monitoring. The knowledge base is unchanged. The available resources are not. This is why capable, well-prepared students sometimes perform below their level and blank despite extensive study. The challenge is often not acquiring more knowledge. Sometimes it is preserving access to knowledge that already exists.

What Helps

Pressure cannot be eliminated completely, nor should it be. Some degree of activation and concern is a natural response to meaningful challenges. Becoming indifferent to performance is neither the goal nor possible.

The goal is to reduce the working memory consumed by worry.

One approach supported by research involves expressive writing before performance situations. Spending a few minutes writing down concerns and worries appears to reduce the cognitive burden associated with carrying those thoughts internally. In a classroom study, students who wrote briefly about their worries shortly before an exam performed better under pressure than those who did not (Ramirez & Beilock, 2011). Rather than repeatedly revisiting concerns during the examination, students have already given those concerns a place to go.

The technique is simple, but its value comes from a deeper principle. Thoughts that continuously compete for attention consume resources. Thoughts that have been acknowledged and externalized often become less demanding.

Eliminating anxiety is not the objective. The objective is to keep anxiety from occupying the space reasoning requires.

Try This Today

What to do: In the few minutes before a high-stakes test, write down your worries about it, plainly and privately, for three or four minutes. Do not try to solve them or argue with them. Set the page aside and begin.

What you may notice: The worry loop quiets enough to free attention for the questions themselves.

Why it matters: Anxious thoughts occupy the same working memory the exam needs. Putting them on paper gives them somewhere to go, which is why brief expressive writing before a test can protect performance (Ramirez & Beilock, 2011).

Relabel the Signal

Under pressure, the body produces a familiar set of signals: a faster heart, shallow breath, a tightening stomach. Students often read these as evidence that something is going wrong, that they are falling apart or unprepared. That reading tends to make the interference worse.

There is a more accurate reading. The same signals are what the body produces when it mobilizes for a demanding task. Relabeling them that way, as *this is my body getting ready, not failing*, improves performance under evaluation, in testing and in public speaking, more reliably than trying to calm down (Jamieson et al., 2012; Jamieson, Mendes,

Blackstock, & Schmader, 2010). A brief version is as simple as telling yourself you are excited rather than anxious before you begin (Brooks, 2014).

This works better than the more common instinct, which is to suppress the feeling. Suppression is effortful and draws on the same working memory the task needs, so it tends to cost performance rather than protect it (Gross, 2002). Reappraisal is cheaper: it changes what the signal means without spending resources fighting it.

The move fits this chapter's account of choking. Blanking under pressure comes partly from attention turned inward to monitor the self, and relabeling arousal as readiness keeps the signal from being read as threat, which frees attention to return to the task. It pairs naturally with the worry-offloading already described (Ramirez & Beilock, 2011): offload the worry onto paper, relabel the arousal as readiness, then begin.

Options Menu

Pressure shows up before a test, during one, and in the body's own signals, and different moments call for different moves. If helpful:

- **Offload on paper before you begin.** For a scheduled, high-stakes test, write the worries out first. It feels unproductive in the moment, and it clears working memory for the task (Ramirez & Beilock, 2011).
- **Reconstruct from one anchor when you blank.** Start from a single fact you are sure of and rebuild outward instead of chasing the whole answer at once. The reach restarts retrieval instead of freezing on the gap.

- **Slow one breath before you answer.** A single deliberate exhale costs a few seconds and pulls arousal down out of the range where retrieval stalls.
- **Rehearse under a little pressure beforehand.** Practice timed, out loud, or standing, closer to exam conditions than silent review. It is less comfortable than quiet practice, and it narrows the gap between practice and performance.
- **Relabel the arousal.** Read the racing heart as your body mobilizing, or tell yourself you are excited. It feels like a trick, and it performs better than trying to calm down (Jamieson et al., 2012; Brooks, 2014).
- **Let the feeling be present.** Suppressing the arousal spends the attention the task needs, so letting the signal sit there costs less than wrestling it (Gross, 2002).

Common Traps

A few responses to a blank moment make the next one more likely.

Reading a blank as proof the knowledge was never there feels like honesty, but a retrieval blank under pressure and a true knowledge gap produce the same silence, and they call for different responses.

Studying the topic harder after a blank assumes more input is the fix. When the failure was arousal narrowing access, additional input leaves the condition that produced it untouched.

Treating the blank as a referendum on belonging turns one taxed moment into a verdict about whether you are cut out for this, which raises arousal the next time the same situation arrives.

Recap

What to hold onto when your mind goes blank:

- **Pressure taxes the working memory retrieval depends on**, so a blank is often a conditions problem rather than a knowledge one.
- **The knowledge usually did not vanish.** The room to reach it narrowed.
- Offloading worry before a test frees attention for the test.
- When you blank, rebuild from one anchor rather than freezing on the whole.
- A blank under pressure is not a verdict on what you know or whether you belong.

Before You Move On

This chapter examined a single pressured moment: knowing something and being unable to reach it when it counts. Pressure does not so much erase knowledge as crowd the working memory that retrieval depends on.

The next chapter widens the lens from the moment to the condition. Anxiety does not only arrive at the exam. It can sit in the room during ordinary studying, changing attention, memory, and how a session is interpreted long before any test begins.

References

Baumeister, R. F. (1984). Choking under pressure: Self-consciousness and paradoxical effects of incentives on skillful performance. *Journal of Personality and Social Psychology, 46*(3), 610–620.

Beilock, S. L., & Carr, T. H. (2005). When high-powered people fail: Working memory and choking under pressure in math. *Psychological Science, 16*(2), 101–105.

Brooks, A. W. (2014). Get excited: Reappraising pre-performance anxiety as excitement. *Journal of Experimental Psychology: General, 143*(3), 1144–1158.

Gross, J. J. (2002). Emotion regulation: Affective, cognitive, and social consequences. *Psychophysiology, 39*(3), 281–291.

Jamieson, J. P., Mendes, W. B., Blackstock, E., & Schmader, T. (2010). Turning the knots in your stomach into bows: Reappraising arousal improves performance on the GRE. *Journal of Experimental Social Psychology, 46*(1), 208–212.

Jamieson, J. P., Nock, M. K., & Mendes, W. B. (2012). Mind over matter: Reappraising arousal improves cardiovascular and cognitive responses to stress. *Journal of Experimental Psychology: General, 141*(3), 417–422.

Ramirez, G., & Beilock, S. L. (2011). Writing about testing worries boosts exam performance in the classroom. *Science, 331*(6014), 211–213.

CHAPTER ELEVEN

When Anxiety Becomes a Learning Problem

Key Question

When does normal stress start interfering with learning itself?

Core Idea

Anxiety becomes a learning problem when it occupies the attention studying requires.

Example Scenario

Imani sits down to study and notices the feeling immediately. Her chest feels tight, her attention keeps drifting, and the list of unfinished work seems larger than it did the night before. Nothing dramatic has happened. There has been no major setback, no failed exam, and no new problem. Yet studying feels different today.

She opens her notes and attempts to focus. After a few minutes she realizes she has reread the same paragraph several times without absorbing it. The harder she tries to concentrate, the more aware she becomes of her difficulty concentrating.

What Imani is running into is a fact about the session, not about herself. Anxiety here works as a learning problem, consuming the attention the studying needs.

Anxiety Is Not Just a Feeling

Students often describe anxiety as if it exists separately from learning. They talk about anxiety on one side and studying on the other, as though the two run independently.

In reality, anxiety affects many of the same systems that learning depends on. Attention becomes more difficult to direct. Working memory becomes easier to overload. Decisions require more effort. Uncertainty becomes harder to tolerate. The same working-memory resources that reasoning and retrieval require can be consumed by managing the feeling itself (Beilock & Carr, 2005).

This matters because students sometimes interpret these changes as evidence that they are becoming less capable. The experience feels like diminished ability, when it is better understood as diminished access to cognitive resources.

The distinction is important because ability and access are not the same thing. A student may possess the necessary knowledge and skills while struggling to use them effectively under conditions of elevated anxiety.

Why Anxiety Consumes Attention

Attention is limited, and anxiety competes for the same resources a study session needs. Concerns about performance and possible failure draw attention that would otherwise go to reading, reasoning, and retrieval, leaving a divided system: part of the mind on the work, part on monitoring threat.

From the inside this feels like an inability to focus. A truer description is that attention is being asked to do two jobs at once. The trouble is not a lack of effort. The effort is real, and it is being distributed across competing demands.

When Anxiety Becomes Evidence

One reason anxiety becomes so disruptive is that students often treat it as information.

Feeling anxious before an exam may be interpreted as evidence that preparation is inadequate. Feeling uncertain during studying may be interpreted as evidence that learning is failing. Feeling overwhelmed may be interpreted as evidence that the situation is unmanageable.

These conclusions can intensify anxiety because the feeling itself becomes proof that something is wrong.

The difficulty is that anxiety is not always a reliable indicator of reality. Anxiety reflects perceived threat, not objective threat. The two sometimes overlap, but they are not identical.

A student can feel anxious and still be well prepared. A student can feel uncertain and still be learning effectively. A student can feel overwhelmed while making meaningful progress.

Treating anxiety as information is useful. Treating it as proof is often less helpful.

Why Medical Students Experience So Much Anxiety

Medical education contains many of the conditions that reliably generate anxiety.

The stakes feel high. The workload is substantial. Feedback is frequent. Performance is visible. Uncertainty is unavoidable. Students are regularly asked to function in situations where complete mastery is impossible.

These conditions do not guarantee anxiety, but they create an environment where anxiety becomes understandable.

This observation matters because students often interpret anxiety as a personal weakness. A more accurate interpretation may be that anxiety is a predictable response to an environment filled with uncertainty, evaluation, and responsibility.

Recognizing this does not eliminate anxiety. It does provide context that can reduce the tendency to view anxiety as evidence of inadequacy.

The Cost of Fighting Every Feeling

Many students respond to anxiety by attempting to eliminate it completely. They treat the presence of anxiety as the problem that must be solved before productive work can begin.

This strategy often creates a second struggle layered on top of the first. The student is now managing both the original anxiety and the frustration of having anxiety.

A more realistic goal is often learning how to function with manageable anxiety. Most medical students will experience anxiety at some point during training. Waiting for complete emotional certainty before studying, testing, or performing is rarely practical.

This does not mean severe anxiety should be endured. When anxiety becomes overwhelming, persistent, or significantly impairing, additional support may be appropriate. The point is narrower than that.

Productive learning does not wait for the complete absence of anxiety. It asks only for enough available attention to engage with the task.

Returning to the Task

Anxiety naturally pulls attention toward possible threats. Learning requires attention to return to the work itself.

Students often find it helpful to focus on specific actions instead of broad outcomes. Broad outcomes are difficult to control and easy to worry about. Immediate actions are easier to influence.

Instead of focusing on whether the next exam will go well, a student can focus on the next retrieval exercise. Instead of focusing on class rank, a student can focus on the next practice question. Instead of focusing on an entire semester, a student can focus on the next study block.

This shift does not solve every problem. It does move attention toward aspects of the situation that are more directly connected to learning.

Try This Today

What to do: During your next study session, notice whenever your attention shifts from the task itself to predictions about future outcomes. Write down the prediction, then return attention to the next concrete action required by the task.

What you may notice: Many anxious thoughts involve future events that cannot be resolved in the current moment. The study task often becomes easier to engage with once attention returns to the immediate work.

Why it matters: Anxiety frequently directs attention toward prediction. Learning requires attention for processing, retrieval, and reasoning. Separating the task from the prediction helps preserve some of those resources.

Options Menu

Anxiety rarely yields to a single move. These help keep it from taking over a study session. If helpful:

- **Name it as load.** Label the feeling, *this is anxiety taxing attention*, before deciding what it means. The small move keeps the feeling from being read as evidence about ability.

- **Offload the worry, then start.** Give the concerns a few minutes on paper, as in the previous chapter, before opening your notes (Ramirez & Beilock, 2011).

- **Shrink the entry point.** Choose one concrete first task, small enough that arousal does not block it, as Chapter One described. The small task gets you past the freeze.
- **Separate the task from the prediction.** When attention jumps to the outcome, note the prediction and return to the next concrete action.

Common Traps

A few responses to anxiety quietly make it harder to study.

Treating anxiety as information about competence feels like vigilance, *if I am this worried, something must be wrong*, but anxiety is persuasive precisely because it feels diagnostic, and it fires in manageable situations as readily as in genuine ones.

Trying to think your way calm before starting assumes you must feel ready first. The rumination uses the same attention the studying needs, so the loop deepens the longer the start is postponed.

Pushing harder against a drifting mind treats focus as a matter of will. When the drift is anxiety consuming working memory, more force tends to narrow attention further instead of restoring it.

Recap

What to hold onto when anxiety is in the room:

- **Anxiety is not only a feeling to wait out.** It consumes the attention and working memory studying requires.
- It feels diagnostic, like evidence about ability, and usually is not.

- **Naming it as load**, instead of treating it as truth, keeps it from becoming a verdict.
- Offloading worry and shrinking the first task free attention to begin.
- The task in front of you and the prediction about the future are different things. Work the task.

Before You Move On

The previous chapter looked at why knowledge can become briefly unreachable under pressure. This chapter widened that idea, examining how anxiety changes the conditions learning depends on by competing for attention, raising cognitive demands, and shaping how students read their own experience.

Anxiety is one way emotion reaches into learning. Another is the way a single difficult event becomes a judgment about the person who experienced it. The next chapter examines why academic struggle so often turns personal, and what becomes possible when a setback is investigated rather than treated as evidence about worth.

References

Beilock, S. L., & Carr, T. H. (2005). When high-powered people fail: Working memory and choking under pressure in math. *Psychological Science, 16*(2), 101–105.

Ramirez, G., & Beilock, S. L. (2011). Writing about testing worries boosts exam performance in the classroom. *Science, 331*(6014), 211–213.

CHAPTER TWELVE

Why Struggle Feels Personal

Key Question

Why does difficulty so quickly become a story about who you are?

Core Idea

The explanation you reach for after a setback shapes what you do next, and the harshest one is rarely the most accurate.

Example Scenario

Fatima misses six questions in a row. The questions cover material she studied earlier in the week, and none of them involve topics she completely ignored. As she works through the explanations, she begins to feel a familiar shift. The disappointment from missing the questions starts to expand into something larger.

By the end of the review session, the problem no longer feels like six missed questions. It feels like evidence that she is falling behind, that she is not learning fast enough, and that she may not be capable of handling the demands of medical school.

Fatima's capability is not what that review session measured. What it shows instead is how fast six missed questions became a sentence about the person who missed them.

It helps to separate the two. The event is what happened. The interpretation is the story told about it afterward, and a more useful question can take that story's place.

Why We Look for Explanations

Human beings naturally explain events because explanations help create a sense of order and predictability. When something goes well, we want to know why. When something goes poorly, we want to know why. Attribution research has long described how the explanations people reach for shape the emotions and expectations that follow (Weiner, 1985).

Medical students do the same thing. Every exam score, question block, clerkship evaluation, and study session provides information that seems to require interpretation. The challenge is that explanations often arrive before careful analysis does.

A student struggles to focus and concludes that motivation is the problem. A student misses several questions and concludes that intelligence is the problem. A student falls behind and concludes that discipline is the problem. These explanations can feel convincing because they are immediate and create a clear story about what happened.

Personal explanations are not always wrong. The trouble is that they are often incomplete. When the first explanation becomes the final explanation, other possibilities never receive fair consideration.

The Fastest Explanation Is Not Always the Most Accurate

The previous chapters explored several reasons studying can become difficult. Cognitive load can make starting difficult (Sweller, 1988), retrieval problems can make knowledge inaccessible, familiarity can create an illusion of learning, and poor calibration can distort judgments about progress.

Those explanations describe conditions, mechanisms, and processes that affect learning. None of them require a deficient student. They show that studying can break down for reasons that are real, understandable, and responsive to adjustment.

Yet many students skip over those possibilities and move directly toward personal conclusions. Learning problems become character problems before other explanations receive consideration. This matters because the explanation chosen influences the response that follows.

A student who believes the problem is laziness will likely respond differently than a student who recognizes cognitive overload. A student who believes the problem is inability will likely respond differently than a student who recognizes a retrieval failure. The quality of the explanation shapes the quality of the solution.

Why High Achievers Are Especially Vulnerable

Many medical students arrive with a long history of success. For years, effort produced results, difficult courses were manageable, good grades were expected, and academic competence became part of how they understood themselves.

Medical school changes that experience. Students encounter larger volumes of information, more uncertainty, and more situations where effort does not immediately produce the desired outcome. Experiences that were once uncommon become routine.

For some students, this is the first time they have struggled consistently despite working hard. The unfamiliarity of that struggle can make it difficult to interpret. When success has been normal for years, difficulty can feel like evidence that something fundamental has changed.

A student who has rarely questioned their academic ability may suddenly question it every week. The intensity of the reaction often reflects the importance of the identity being challenged. Beliefs about whether ability is fixed or developed shape how heavily that challenge lands (Dweck, 2006).

When Performance Becomes Identity

Academic performance provides information. A score tells you how you performed on a particular assessment under particular conditions. A question block provides information about what was accessible during that exercise. Feedback identifies strengths and weaknesses.

These sources of information become harmful when they are treated as measures of personal worth. A missed question becomes evidence of incompetence. A poor grade becomes evidence of inadequacy. A difficult semester becomes evidence that a student does not belong.

The interpretation expands beyond the information available. This expansion happens so quickly that many students never notice it occurring. The transition from *I struggled with this task* to *I am struggling as a person* can feel almost automatic.

The trouble is not that students care about performance. It is that performance and identity begin to merge. When that happens, academic information becomes harder to use because it has become emotionally loaded with questions of worth and belonging.

What Gets Lost When Everything Becomes Personal

When every setback becomes evidence about identity, useful questions become harder to ask, and students stop examining conditions to start examining themselves. A difficult session raises one question above the others, *What is wrong with me?*, when the more useful one asks what made the task hard, what skill it tested, and what would make the next attempt more workable. One question encourages judgment. The other encourages investigation, and investigation is what creates room to adjust.

The Difference Between Explanation and Evaluation

Students often treat explanations and evaluations as the same thing, but they are different tasks. An explanation attempts to understand what happened. An evaluation attempts to determine what something means about the student.

Suppose a student performs poorly on an exam. An explanation might consider preparation, retrieval, fatigue, stress, study strategy, question interpretation, or time management. The goal is understanding.

An evaluation asks whether the result reflects positively or negatively on the student. The difficulty arises when evaluation replaces explanation. Instead of understanding the event, the student immediately begins assessing themselves.

The result may be harsh self-criticism, but even positive self-evaluation can interfere with learning if it prevents careful analysis. Understanding usually requires curiosity. Evaluation often ends the investigation before it begins.

Replacing Judgment With Investigation

A calmer response begins with different questions: what happened, what conditions contributed, what skill is being developed, what evidence supports the interpretation. These do not guarantee a comforting answer, and sometimes a student does need to confront a real gap. The point is to reach conclusions through investigation instead of assumption, keeping the possibilities (load, retrieval, fatigue, calibration, unrealistic expectations) visible long enough to be considered before judgment narrows them.

What You Would Tell Someone Else

Many students apply a standard to themselves that they would never apply to another student. A classmate misses several questions and receives understanding. The same student misses several questions and receives criticism.

A friend struggles after a difficult week and receives compassion. The same struggle in oneself becomes evidence of inadequacy. This difference is worth noticing because it often reveals how quickly students move from observation to judgment.

The point is consistency, not reassurance. If an explanation seems unreasonable when applied to another capable student, it may deserve closer examination when applied to yourself.

Try This Today

What to do: After a difficult study session, exam, or question block, write down your first explanation. Then generate three additional explanations that do not involve character, intelligence, or worth.

What you may notice: The first explanation often focuses on personal deficiency. Additional explanations frequently include factors that were initially overlooked, such as task design, fatigue, retrieval conditions, unclear priorities, or unrealistic expectations.

Why it matters: The goal is to consider a wider range of explanations before deciding what happened, with personal responsibility still on the table.

Options Menu

When a setback starts hardening into a judgment, these are ways to investigate instead of evaluate. If helpful:

- **Generate three non-character explanations.** Name three that do not involve intelligence, worth, or discipline before accepting the first story. It takes effort when you are discouraged, and it keeps the personal explanation from being the only one on the table.
- **Apply the consistency test.** Ask what you would conclude if a capable classmate described this exact experience. It can feel like

letting yourself off the hook, and it is actually holding one standard instead of two.

- **Name the condition, then the fix.** Tie the difficulty to a mechanism (load, access, fatigue, format) and let that point to the response. It is slower than a verdict, and verdicts do not come with next steps.

Common Traps

The move from a learning problem to a character problem happens fast, and a few habits speed it up.

Reaching for the fastest explanation gives you an immediate story, and in a high-achieving person the fastest story is usually a personal one. It feels like accountability while quietly closing off the more accurate, more fixable explanations.

Letting evaluation replace investigation feels like seriousness, *I should be hard on myself about this*, but evaluation ends the inquiry before it starts, and harsh self-judgment produces distress instead of a plan.

Applying a standard to yourself you would never apply to a peer guarantees the conclusion about you is harsher than the evidence supports.

Recap

What to hold onto when a setback starts to feel personal:

- **A learning problem becomes a character problem quickly,** and the speed is the thing to watch.

- **The first explanation is usually personal**, and usually incomplete.
- **Investigation asks what made this hard.** Evaluation asks what it says about you. Only the first creates a next move.
- A standard you would not apply to a classmate probably should not apply to you.
- Naming the condition turns a verdict back into a problem you can act on.

Before You Move On

This chapter turned to interpretation, examining how a learning problem becomes a judgment about the person who has it.

Struggle often feels personal because academic difficulties are easy to transform into stories about identity. The interpretation can feel obvious even when it is incomplete. Learning becomes easier to understand when events are investigated before they are evaluated.

Even when students learn to interpret setbacks more carefully, another challenge remains. Medical training places students in constant contact with the performance of other capable people. The next chapter examines comparison, why it becomes so powerful in medical education, and how it can distort judgments about progress, ability, and belonging.

References

Dweck, C. S. (2006). *Mindset: The new psychology of success.* Random House.

Sweller, J. (1988). Cognitive load during problem solving: Effects on learning. *Cognitive Science, 12*(2), 257–285.

Weiner, B. (1985). An attributional theory of achievement motivation and emotion. *Psychological Review, 92*(4), 548–573.

CHAPTER THIRTEEN

Unsettled Is Not Unprepared

Key Question

Why can you feel behind even when you are keeping up?

Core Idea

Feeling unsettled often reflects comparison and belonging more than how prepared you are.

Example Scenario

Connor leaves a lecture feeling unsettled.

The material was difficult, but that is not what bothers him. What stays with him is a conversation he overheard while packing up his laptop. Several classmates were discussing practice questions, and they seemed to understand concepts that still felt confusing to him.

On the drive home, Connor stops thinking about the lecture itself. Instead, he begins thinking about everyone else. They seem more prepared. They seem more confident. They seem less overwhelmed.

By the end of the evening, Connor is no longer evaluating his own learning. He is evaluating himself relative to other people.

Where Connor stands is not something a drive home can settle. The telling part is the shift: he stopped evaluating his own learning and started evaluating himself against people whose inner experience he cannot see.

Why Comparison Feels Useful

Comparison exists for a reason.

People often understand their progress by observing others. In unfamiliar situations, comparison can provide information about expectations, standards, and performance (Festinger, 1954).

Medical school creates many opportunities for this process. Students compare exam scores, study schedules, clinical evaluations, research productivity, board preparation, and career plans. These comparisons can sometimes provide useful information.

A student may discover a study strategy worth trying. Another may realize that a particular struggle is more common than expected. Comparison can occasionally increase perspective and reduce isolation.

The trouble is not that students compare themselves to others. It is that the information available for comparison is often incomplete.

The Visibility Problem

Students have direct access to their own struggles and only partial access to everyone else's.

You know when you feel confused. You know how often you change answers, how much material you forgot, how many questions you missed, and how uncertain you feel.

Most of that information remains invisible in other people.

Instead, students often see polished outcomes. They see high scores, confident comments, successful presentations, and completed projects. The private uncertainty behind those outcomes is much harder to observe.

This creates an uneven comparison. Students compare their internal experience to other people's external presentation. The comparison feels fair because both sides appear visible. In reality, one side contains substantially more information than the other.

The result is predictable. Many students conclude that they are struggling more than everyone else because they possess evidence of their own difficulties and relatively little evidence of anyone else's.

The Myth of the Effortless Student

Every medical school seems to have a student who appears effortlessly competent: quick with answers, calm before exams, fluent with the material. It is tempting to read that surface as evidence that some people simply belong more naturally in medicine.

The story is built from incomplete information. What stays invisible is the time that student spends studying, the anxiety they carry, the questions they miss in private, the doubt they do not show. Differences in ability are real, but the effortless surface usually hides a process much like everyone else's.

Comparison Changes the Meaning of Progress

One of the most frustrating effects of comparison is that it can make genuine progress feel insignificant.

A student improves from passing practice questions half the time to passing them three-quarters of the time. Viewed independently, that is meaningful improvement.

The emotional impact changes when comparison enters the picture. If classmates appear to be performing even better, the student's attention shifts away from progress and toward relative position.

The result is that improvement stops feeling like improvement.

Medical education already provides many objective challenges. Comparison adds a second challenge by changing how students interpret their own development. Progress becomes harder to appreciate when every gain is immediately evaluated against someone else's performance.

Why Comparison Intensifies During Uncertainty

Comparison tends to become stronger when students feel uncertain.

When people are confident about where they stand, they often rely more heavily on their own observations. When uncertainty increases, outside information becomes more appealing.

Medical education contains a great deal of uncertainty. Students are constantly learning new material, adapting to unfamiliar expectations, and receiving feedback that may be difficult to interpret.

Under those conditions, comparison can feel like a shortcut to understanding performance.

The difficulty is that comparison rarely resolves uncertainty as effectively as students hope. Instead, it often replaces one uncertainty with another. Instead of wondering how they are doing, students begin wondering how they compare.

Those are different questions. Only one of them directly improves learning.

The Hidden Cost of Upward Comparison

Students often compare themselves to people who appear to be performing better.

Psychologists refer to this as upward comparison (Buunk & Gibbons, 2007). Sometimes it can be motivating. A student may learn from a peer's approach or become inspired by what seems possible.

The benefits are usually discussed more often than the costs.

Upward comparison can distort perceptions of normal progress. It can create unrealistic expectations about how quickly learning should occur. It can also make students overlook evidence of their own growth because attention remains focused elsewhere.

When comparison becomes constant, students may begin treating exceptional performance as the standard against which everything should be measured. That standard is difficult to maintain because it is often based on a selective sample of highly visible successes.

Returning Attention to the Actual Task

Comparison and isolation are not the only options.

Students benefit from learning from peers, sharing strategies, and supporting one another. The goal is to return attention to the task that actually matters, which does not require ignoring other people.

Learning depends on whether knowledge is becoming more accessible, understanding is becoming deeper, and skills are becoming more reliable. Those questions can be answered without knowing how another student performed.

Comparison becomes less powerful when students return to evidence that is directly connected to their own development. A few questions tend to help: whether you can retrieve material more reliably than before, whether a concept is clearer than it was last week, whether the mistakes you make now differ from the ones you made a month ago, and what specific skill you are trying to improve. These focus attention on growth instead of ranking.

Comparison and Belonging

Many students assume that comparison is mainly about performance. Often it is also about belonging. Belonging carries real weight in medical training. Research on why students persist or leave has found that a sense of academic and social connection is among the stronger predictors of whether they continue (Tinto, 1993).

Students look around the room and try to determine whether they fit. They wonder whether their struggles are normal, whether their uncertainty is acceptable, and whether they belong among people who appear more confident.

The challenge is that belonging cannot be accurately measured through observation alone. People tend to overestimate how visible their own nervousness is and how much others are scrutinizing them (Gilovich et al., 2000), which makes another student's calm look like proof of belonging it cannot really provide.

The students who seem most confident may have many of the same concerns. The students who appear calm may be managing substantial uncertainty. The students who look comfortable may be questioning themselves more than anyone realizes.

Comparison often creates the illusion that everyone else is adapting more successfully. That illusion becomes more convincing when nobody talks openly about the parts of training that feel difficult.

Try This Today

What to do: Choose one area of studying that currently feels discouraging. Instead of comparing yourself to another student, compare your current performance to where you were three months ago.

What you may notice: The comparison often reveals progress that was previously overlooked. Skills that still feel incomplete may be substantially stronger than they once were.

Why it matters: Improvement is easier to recognize when the reference point reflects your own development instead of someone else's performance.

Options Menu

Comparison is hard to switch off, and these make it less distorting. If helpful:

- **Compare to your past self.** Set today's performance beside where you were a few months ago instead of beside a classmate. It is less immediate than ranking, and it measures development instead of position.

- **Name what you cannot see.** When a classmate looks effortless, list the invisible inputs: a prior elective, private hours, hidden uncertainty. It can feel like rationalizing, and it corrects a genuinely uneven comparison.

- **Turn comparison into a question.** Convert *they are ahead of me* into *what are they doing that I could try?* It requires swallowing the sting, and it extracts the one useful thing comparison offers.

- **Return to task evidence.** Ask whether your own retrieval, understanding, and errors are improving. These are questions you can answer without reference to anyone else.

Common Traps

Comparison misleads in a few reliable ways.

Comparing your inside to someone else's outside feels fair because both performances seem visible, but you hold full evidence of your own struggle and almost none of theirs, so the comparison is uneven before it starts.

Treating the most visible successes as the standard quietly sets the bar at a selective sample of other people's best moments, against which ordinary progress always looks like falling behind.

Reading other students' calm as evidence they belong more than you mistakes a surface for the whole. The students who look most settled are often managing the same uncertainty.

Recap

What to hold onto when everyone else seems further ahead:

- **Comparison runs on uneven information: all of your struggle,** little of theirs.
- **The effortless student is a surface.** The hours, the misses, and the doubt behind it are rarely visible.
- **Comparison grows under uncertainty and seldom resolves it,** swapping *how am I doing?* for *how do I compare?*
- **The reference point that tracks learning is your past self.** The person beside you is the wrong yardstick.
- Progress stops feeling like progress the moment it is graded against someone else's best moments.

Before You Move On

The previous chapter explored why learning problems often become identity judgments. This chapter examined how comparison amplifies them, supplying a steady stream of information about other people's performance that is easy to misread.

Setbacks and comparison are sharpest in a single moment. The next chapter turns to time. It examines why a hard week can feel as though it undoes months of work, and how stress that accumulates slowly shapes the way a single difficult stretch is experienced.

References

Buunk, A. P., & Gibbons, F. X. (2007). Social comparison: The end of a theory and the emergence of a field. *Organizational Behavior and Human Decision Processes, 102*(1), 3–21.

Festinger, L. (1954). A theory of social comparison processes. *Human Relations, 7*(2), 117–140.

Gilovich, T., Medvec, V. H., & Savitsky, K. (2000). The spotlight effect in social judgment. *Current Directions in Psychological Science, 9*(1), 1–4.

Tinto, V. (1993). *Leaving college: Rethinking the causes and cures of student attrition* (2nd ed.). University of Chicago Press.

CHAPTER FOURTEEN

Why One Hard Week Feels Like It Undoes Everything

Key Question

Why can one hard week feel like proof that everything is falling apart?

Core Idea

A hard week usually lands on accumulated strain, so the reaction reflects the buildup more than the week.

Example Scenario

Hana cannot point to anything dramatic. The week was ordinary (one more deadline, one more short night), yet it has flattened her in a way that seems out of proportion, and she finds herself wondering *why am I handling an ordinary week so poorly?*

Reading Hana's week on its own is exactly the misreading this chapter is about. The week is not the whole story: it landed on months of accumulated load, and the size of her response fits the total, not the final straw.

Looking at the Wrong Time Scale

When students begin struggling, they often search for a recent explanation. They ask themselves what happened this week, what happened yesterday, or what happened during the last examination. The assumption is that a noticeable symptom should have a recent cause.

Sometimes that is true. More often, the explanation extends much further back.

A student may notice increasing difficulty concentrating during lectures. Another may find that studying feels unusually effortful. Someone else may become more irritable, emotionally exhausted, or discouraged by challenges that previously felt manageable. Because the change feels recent, students often attribute it to whatever happened most recently.

The mind naturally searches for immediate causes. The body, however, often keeps a longer record.

Stress researchers Bruce McEwen and John Wingfield argued that the cumulative burden of repeated demands may matter more than any individual event (McEwen & Wingfield, 2003). A difficult week is rarely experienced in isolation. It arrives within the context of everything that preceded it.

Why the Small Stuff Suddenly Feels Heavy

McEwen described this cumulative process using the concept of allostatic load. The term refers to the wear and tear that accumulates when the body and mind must repeatedly adapt to ongoing demands without sufficient opportunities for recovery (McEwen, 1998).

Adaptation itself is not the problem. Human beings are remarkably capable of responding to challenges. Students routinely adjust to difficult schedules, examinations, changing clinical environments, and high expectations.

Problems emerge when adaptation becomes continuous.

A single night of inadequate sleep is usually manageable. A single stressful examination is usually manageable. A difficult conversation with a supervisor is usually manageable. Most students can absorb these experiences and continue functioning effectively.

Months of disrupted sleep, persistent uncertainty, frequent evaluation, emotional strain, and sustained vigilance create something different. The individual stressor is no longer the challenge. The cumulative load generated by repeated adaptation is.

This distinction helps explain why students sometimes feel surprised by their own reactions. The final stressor appears relatively small, yet the response feels disproportionately large. What looks like an overreaction may actually reflect the accumulated effects of many previous demands.

Why Burnout Builds Gradually

Students often describe burnout as if it arrived unexpectedly.

One day everything seemed manageable. Then, seemingly without warning, motivation disappeared, concentration declined, and emotional exhaustion became difficult to ignore.

The experience feels sudden because awareness often arrives late. The underlying process is usually much slower.

A student may spend months functioning under increasing levels of strain. Sleep becomes slightly less restorative. Recovery periods become shorter. Emotional reserves become thinner. Small frustrations require greater effort to manage. None of these changes feels dramatic enough to demand attention.

Because adaptation occurs gradually, the cumulative burden can remain largely invisible until functioning begins to noticeably decline.

When symptoms eventually become difficult to ignore, students often search for a single explanation. They focus on the most recent examination, the most recent rotation, or the most recent disappointment. While those events may contribute, they are often only the final additions to a much larger load that has been accumulating over time.

Burnout rarely emerges from one difficult day. More often, it emerges from a prolonged mismatch between demands and recovery.

When Students Blame Themselves

One consequence of misunderstanding cumulative stress is that students frequently interpret stress-related symptoms as personal failures.

Difficulty concentrating may be interpreted as laziness. Emotional exhaustion may be interpreted as insufficient resilience. Reduced cognitive efficiency may be interpreted as a lack of discipline. Irritability may be interpreted as a character flaw.

These explanations feel plausible because the symptoms are experienced internally. Students assume the problem must originate within themselves.

The research on stress suggests a broader perspective. Difficulty concentrating, emotional exhaustion, increased irritability, and reduced mental efficiency are not always signs of insufficient effort. In many cases, they are signs that the system has been carrying too much load for too long.

This distinction does not eliminate responsibility. Students still benefit from examining their habits, decisions, and coping strategies. The important point is that not every decline in performance reflects a deficit of motivation or character.

Sometimes the issue is cumulative strain. The response required in those situations may be different from simply trying harder.

Recovery Is Part of Performance

Medical culture often treats recovery as separate from achievement, an interruption to productivity. The physiology of stress suggests otherwise: recovery is one of the mechanisms that lets adaptation continue, and without restoration the systems behind attention, emotional regulation, memory, and decision-making become harder to sustain.

This is counterintuitive to ambitious students. When performance slips, the instinct is to add hours. Sometimes that is right. At other times the limiting factor is recovery, not effort, and added demand only produces diminishing returns, working harder while accomplishing less. The goal is not less ambition. It is recognizing that recovery and performance work together.

The Invisible Nature of Accumulation

Because adaptation is gradual, it can mask deterioration. Students grow accustomed to fatigue and sustained pressure the way people grow used to background noise. A student running at eighty percent of their usual capacity may not notice the change, and someone sleeping poorly for months may treat constant fatigue as normal.

This makes self-assessment hard, because students compare their current state to their recent past instead of to a healthier baseline. Cumulative strain stays hidden until functioning drops far enough to force attention.

A Quick Load-and-Recovery Check

Because accumulated load is hard to see from the inside, a periodic check helps. None of these is conclusive on its own. Taken together, they suggest whether demand has been outrunning recovery:

- Is sleep shorter or more broken than it was a month ago?
- Are small frustrations landing harder than they used to?
- Has concentration or recall slipped across the board instead of on a single topic?
- When was the last genuinely unhurried stretch of recovery, and how long ago?

- Is the reaction to the latest week out of proportion to the week itself?

If several point the same way, the useful next move is usually recovery instead of more hours.

Understanding this tendency can help students recognize that adaptation and well-being are not always the same thing. The ability to continue functioning does not necessarily mean that recovery needs are being met.

Try This Today

What to do: When a reaction feels out of proportion to the week, sketch the past few months instead of the past few days. Note sleep, demands, recovery, and any larger stressors, then locate this week on that longer curve.

What you may notice: The response usually fits the accumulated load, even when it looks like an overreaction to the week alone.

Why it matters: The mind reaches for a recent cause while the body keeps a longer record. Reading the longer timeline turns *why am I handling this so poorly?* into a more accurate question about how much has built up and how little recovery has kept pace.

Options Menu

When a week lands harder than it should, these help you respond to the load instead of the last straw. If helpful:

- **Map the longer timeline.** Locate the week on the past few months before deciding what the reaction means.

- **Run a Minimum Viable Day.** On the most depleted days, hold a small, defined unit of study instead of pushing for a normal load (see Chapter Twenty-Two).
- **Protect one recovery window.** Defend a single reliable period of genuine rest instead of waiting for a clear stretch that never quite comes.
- **Check demand against recovery.** When capacity is dropping, ask whether the limiting factor is effort or recovery before adding more hours.

Common Traps

A few readings of a hard week make it harder to interpret.

Searching only the recent past for the cause assumes a visible symptom has a recent source. Cumulative strain builds slowly and stays invisible until function drops, so the latest week takes blame that belongs to months.

Reading stress symptoms as character flaws treats poor concentration, irritability, and exhaustion as evidence of weak discipline, when they are often signs of a system carrying too much for too long.

Answering declining capacity with more hours assumes effort is always the lever. When recovery is the limiting factor, added demand produces diminishing returns instead of more learning.

Recap

What to hold onto when one hard week feels like too much:

- Stress is cumulative, and the burden of repeated adaptation matters more than any single week.
- A response that looks disproportionate to the week often fits the months behind it.
- **Burnout usually develops gradually.** The buildup is slow and awareness comes late.
- Concentration loss, irritability, and exhaustion can be load signals instead of character flaws.
- **When recovery cannot keep pace with demand**, the answer is recovery, not more effort.

Before You Move On

This chapter looked at stress as something that accumulates, and at why a single hard week can carry the weight of the months beneath it. The response those situations call for is often recovery, not more effort.

The next chapter stays with recovery and examines it directly. Learning runs on a biological system with real limits, and sleep, fatigue, and rest shape what attention and memory can do, which makes recovery part of performance instead of a pause from it.

Minimum Viable Day

On a depleted day, the aim is to keep the system running instead of hitting a normal target. A Minimum Viable Day is a smaller, defined unit of study, chosen in advance, that holds continuity without deepening the deficit. A single question set and one topic reviewed can be enough to keep momentum while the load comes down. The fuller version appears in Chapter Twenty-Two. Here it is the practical companion to recognizing accumulated load.

References

McEwen, B. S. (1998). Protective and damaging effects of stress mediators. *New England Journal of Medicine, 338*(3), 171–179.

McEwen, B. S., & Wingfield, J. C. (2003). The concept of allostasis in biology and biomedicine. *Hormones and Behavior, 43*(1), 2–15.

CHAPTER FIFTEEN

Recovery Is Part of Learning

Key Question

Is rest taken away from studying, or part of how it works?

Core Idea

Sleep, rest, and recovery set the capacity everything else in studying depends on.

Example Scenario

Noah decides to push through.

The exam is approaching, the workload is growing, and there never seems to be enough time. He begins sleeping less, taking fewer breaks, and extending study sessions later into the night. The decision feels responsible because it appears to create more time for learning.

For a few days, the strategy seems to work. More material gets covered, more flashcards get reviewed, and more hours are spent studying. The additional effort feels productive because the increase in activity is easy to observe.

As the week continues, something changes. Concentration becomes more difficult. Simple decisions require more effort. Reading slows down. Retrieval becomes less reliable. Noah responds by studying even longer because he assumes the problem is insufficient effort.

Plenty of students hit a stretch like Noah's, where the dip has nothing to do with commitment. The trap is in the pattern: performance fell, he read it as too little effort, and added the one thing, lost recovery, that was driving the fall.

Learning Happens in a Biological System

Students often think about learning as a cognitive process.

They focus on memory, attention, retrieval, understanding, and problem-solving. These processes are important, but they do not operate independently of the body.

Attention depends on biological resources. Memory depends on biological resources. Decision-making depends on biological resources. Every cognitive process discussed in this book occurs within a nervous system that has limits.

These limits are easy to forget because they are always present. Students become accustomed to functioning while tired, stressed, and overloaded. Over time, those conditions can begin to feel normal.

The trouble is that normal and optimal are not the same thing. A student can adapt to chronic fatigue while still experiencing meaningful reductions in learning efficiency.

Understanding this distinction helps explain why effort sometimes produces diminishing returns.

Sleep Does More Than Prevent Exhaustion

Many students think about sleep primarily in terms of energy.

Sleep certainly affects how alert a person feels during the day. The relationship between sleep and learning extends beyond alertness.

Research suggests that sleep contributes to memory consolidation, the process through which newly learned information becomes more stable and accessible over time (Diekelmann & Born, 2010). Learning does not end when a study session ends. Some of the work continues afterward.

This observation creates an important tension for students. Staying awake longer creates more time available for studying. Sleeping creates conditions that support the retention of what was studied.

The tradeoff is not always obvious in the moment because the benefits of additional studying are visible immediately, while the benefits of sleep often become apparent later.

Students do not need perfect sleep to learn effectively. The broader point is that sleep can be part of how learning consolidates.

Fatigue Changes More Than Energy

Fatigue is often described as a lack of energy.

The experience is usually more complicated than that. Fatigue influences attention, working memory, decision-making, emotional regulation, and motivation, and even short-term sleep loss has measurable effects across these areas (Lim & Dinges, 2010).

A tired student may interpret these changes as evidence of poor focus or declining discipline. In some situations, fatigue provides a simpler explanation.

Tasks feel larger when attention is depleted. Retrieval becomes more difficult when cognitive resources are reduced. Emotional reactions often become stronger when fatigue is present.

These effects can create misleading conclusions. A student may assume they have lost motivation when they are actually exhausted. Another may assume they are becoming less capable when they are functioning under conditions of reduced recovery.

This does not mean every struggle is caused by fatigue. It means fatigue deserves consideration before broader conclusions are reached.

Why Stress Feels Different Over Time

Stress is not always harmful.

Short periods of stress can increase focus, direct attention, and mobilize effort. Many students have experienced situations where a deadline or challenge temporarily improved performance.

The difficulty emerges when stress becomes prolonged.

Chronic stress affects multiple systems throughout the body. When activation becomes persistent, the costs begin to accumulate (Sapolsky, 2004).

Students often notice these costs indirectly. Concentration becomes less reliable. Recovery becomes less complete. Small setbacks produce larger emotional reactions. Tasks that once felt manageable begin to feel heavier.

The experience can be confusing because students continue working hard. From their perspective, nothing about their commitment has changed. The conditions supporting that effort may have changed substantially.

The Productivity Illusion

Many students assume that more hours automatically produce more learning.

The assumption feels reasonable because time matters. Learning requires effort, and effort requires time. The relationship between time and learning is not perfectly linear.

An additional hour of focused studying may be highly productive. An additional hour added to the end of an already exhausted day may produce far less learning than expected.

This observation is important because students often evaluate study plans primarily by quantity. The focus becomes how many hours were spent instead of the conditions under which those hours occurred.

Quality and quantity both matter. Ignoring either one creates an incomplete picture.

Recovery Supports Performance

Recovery is often treated as a reward earned after the work is done. Medical education makes that understandable: the work feels endless, so recovery gets postponed to a point that never quite arrives.

A clearer way to see recovery is as part of performance. Sleep supports consolidation, breaks restore attention, physical activity supports mood and cognition, and time away lowers the load carried into the next session. None of these replace studying. They create the conditions under which studying works.

The Difference Between Capacity and Commitment

When students struggle, they often evaluate commitment first.

They ask whether they care enough, whether they are trying hard enough, or whether they are disciplined enough. Those questions can be useful in some situations. They can also obscure another possibility.

A student may be fully committed while operating near the limits of available capacity. The issue is not willingness. It is that biological and cognitive systems have finite resources.

This distinction appeared earlier in the discussion of cognitive load. Capacity influences learning regardless of how motivated a person feels.

Recognizing limits does not lower expectations. It helps students make decisions that align effort with available resources.

Sustainable Learning Requires Sustainability

Medical students often think in terms of individual days.

A difficult exam, a demanding week, or an approaching deadline can dominate attention. These events matter, but learning occurs across months and years, not individual evenings.

Strategies that are effective for a short period may become less effective when sustained indefinitely.

A study plan that consistently sacrifices sleep may eventually reduce the quality of learning. A schedule that leaves no room for recovery may increase vulnerability to fatigue and burnout.

Comfort is not the goal. Medical training will remain demanding. Sustainability is. Learning systems work best when they can continue functioning over time. When fatigue, low mood, or exhaustion become persistent or severe, they call for more than a study adjustment. Recovery and well-being are taken up more fully in the companion volumes of this series, and institutional support services exist for exactly these moments.

Try This Today

What to do: For one week, pay attention to the relationship between recovery and studying. Notice how concentration, retrieval, and decision-making change after nights of better sleep, periods of recovery, or extended fatigue.

What you may notice: Performance often fluctuates alongside recovery more than students expect. Some study problems that appear motivational may have a substantial physiological component.

Why it matters: Recovery influences the conditions under which learning occurs. Understanding those conditions makes it easier to interpret performance accurately.

Options Menu

Recovery is easy to treat as optional, and these keep it inside the work. If helpful:

- **Check recovery before adding hours.** When performance dips, check sleep and load before concluding the problem is effort or that motivation failed.
- **Protect the sleep around heavy study.** Treat the night after a demanding session as part of the studying, since consolidation continues there (Diekelmann & Born, 2010).
- **Run a Minimum Viable Day when depleted.** Hold a small, defined unit instead of a full load on the worst days (see Chapter Twenty-Two).

Common Traps

Recovery gets squeezed out by a few reasonable-sounding beliefs.

Treating recovery as a reward earned after the work assumes rest must be deserved. In a field where the work never ends, that logic postpones recovery indefinitely and erodes the conditions performance depends on.

Counting hours as the measure of a study plan ignores the condition those hours occurred under. An hour added to an exhausted day is not the hour it looks like on the tally.

Reading a capacity problem as a commitment problem assumes trying harder is always available. When the limit is biological, *try harder* asks more of the system that is already depleted.

Recap

What to hold onto when more effort stops producing more learning:

- **Learning runs on a biological system with real limits**, and normal and optimal are not the same.
- **Sleep can support learning by consolidating it**, so it is part of studying instead of time taken from it.
- Fatigue changes attention, retrieval, and emotion, and deserves consideration before harsher explanations.
- **Recovery is a component of performance**, not a reward that follows it.
- What works for a single week can fail across a year, and sustainable learning needs sustainability.

Before You Move On

The previous chapter looked at how stress accumulates over months. This chapter examined the biological systems beneath attention, memory, and performance, and why recovery belongs inside the work rather than after it.

The chapters so far have stayed close to the individual learner: load, access, strategy, emotion, and recovery. Learning also happens somewhere, inside training environments that carry their own expectations, feedback, and culture. The next part turns to those systems, and to how much of what feels personal is shaped by the setting in which it occurs.

References

Diekelmann, S., & Born, J. (2010). The memory function of sleep. *Nature Reviews Neuroscience, 11*(2), 114–126.

Lim, J., & Dinges, D. F. (2010). A meta-analysis of the impact of short-term sleep deprivation on cognitive variables. *Psychological Bulletin, 136*(3), 375–389.

Sapolsky, R. M. (2004). *Why zebras don't get ulcers* (3rd ed.). Holt.

PART FOUR

Learning Inside the System

By this point, many of the explanations students reach for have been examined from a different angle. Cognitive overload can make studying hard to enter. Retrieval failures can look like learning failures. Anxiety, comparison, and self-judgment can change how performance is read. Recovery and capacity shape what effort is able to accomplish.

Those chapters stayed close to the individual learner. This part widens the frame.

Medical students do not learn in a vacuum. They learn inside environments (clinical teams, evaluation structures, institutional cultures) that shape what learning feels like and how students interpret themselves within it. Much of what feels personal is partly a response to these conditions.

The chapters here move from the largest of those conditions to the smallest. Chapter Sixteen examines what changes when learning becomes public, as it does on the wards, where thinking happens in view and education can no longer be cleanly separated from performance. Chapter Seventeen turns to the systems themselves: the hidden curriculum, the unevenness of feedback, and the culture that shapes how the same event is interpreted. Chapter Eighteen narrows all the way down to a single task a student cannot begin, and examines avoidance as a response to the conditions surrounding the work rather than a failure of will.

Together, these chapters move attention from the learner alone to the settings that determine what learning feels like and whether effort can do its work.

CHAPTER SIXTEEN

Learning in Public

Key Question

Why do the clinical years feel so exposing even when you are learning well?

Core Idea

Knowledge now develops in view of others, which changes how learning feels without changing your ability.

Example Scenario

Marcus is asked to present his patient on morning rounds. He has the facts, but halfway through the assessment his reasoning falters, the attending is watching, and he can feel his differential coming apart in front of everyone. Afterward, he is certain he has just shown the whole team how little he knows.

The discomfort Marcus feels on that presentation is not a gauge of how far behind he is. What changed is the setting he is learning in. Knowledge that used to develop in private is now developing in full view, which is much of what makes the clinical years feel exposing.

What Progress Actually Looks Like

It helps to have a map of the path itself. Studying how clinicians develop, Patricia Benner described skill growing through stages, moving from novice, who leans on explicit rules and guidance, through advanced beginner and competent, to proficient and finally expert, where judgment becomes fluid and pattern-based (Benner, 1984). Two features of that progression matter on the wards. Movement through the stages comes from experience in real situations, not from accumulating more facts. And the early stages are meant to feel rule-bound, effortful, and uncertain, because that is what working without a deep store of recognized patterns feels like. A student who feels like a novice on a new rotation is standing at the start of a known trajectory. On this map, uncertainty is a stage to move through, and the early awkwardness is part of how expertise gets built.

Observation alone turns out to be insufficient. Watching experienced clinicians reveals patterns, language, and approaches that would otherwise stay invisible, but many parts of medicine become clear only through participation: a presentation is understood differently when you must deliver it, a differential when you must defend it, a difficult conversation when you must navigate it instead of watching (Irby, 1995). Participation is what turns knowledge into capability.

For many students, the clinical years also involve a shift in identity. Individuals who were accustomed to feeling knowledgeable suddenly find themselves surrounded by professionals with far greater experience. Questions that once seemed straightforward become complicated. Conditions that appeared simple in textbooks reveal layers of nuance and uncertainty. The experience can be humbling, particularly for students whose earlier educational success was built on being well prepared.

Yet humility is not necessarily a sign of diminished competence. It may instead reflect a more accurate understanding of the complexity of clinical work. The student who recognizes how much remains to be learned is often seeing medicine more clearly than before.

Learning in public is rarely comfortable. Most people would rather show finished products than unfinished thinking, and clinical education asks for the opposite. The central challenge of the clinical years is to become more capable through repeated engagement with real clinical work, not to appear finished. Students learn medicine by participating in medicine, and the process is often imperfect, sometimes humbling, and one of the main ways clinical expertise begins to develop.

Try This Today

What to do: The next time you are asked something on rounds and you are not sure, say what you do think and where your reasoning runs out, instead of waiting until you are certain. *My leading diagnosis is X, because of A and B. What I cannot yet account for is C.*

What you may notice: The discussion that follows a partial answer is usually more useful than a polished one would have been, and the discomfort fades faster than expected.

Why it matters: Supervisors can teach to your reasoning only when they can see it. Putting unfinished thinking into words is how clinical reasoning gets corrected and built.

A few phrasings help you stay in the conversation when you are unsure: *My leading diagnosis is ___, because of ___, and what I can't yet explain is ___. I'm not certain, but here is how I'm reasoning through it. I don't know that one. How would you approach it?*

Options Menu

Participating before you feel ready is the skill the clinical years ask for. Ways to make that easier:

- **Offer a tentative hypothesis.** Commit to a leading answer and your reasoning, then invite correction. It risks being wrong out loud, and it gives your thinking somewhere to be improved.

- **Name the part you're unsure of.** Present what you know and mark the gap explicitly. It feels exposing, and it directs the teaching to where you need it.

- **Ask the question you're avoiding.** When something is unclear, ask in the moment instead of resolving to look it up later. It costs a little pride and usually saves a misunderstanding.

- **Treat the correction as the lesson.** When your reasoning is adjusted, record what changed, not only that you were wrong. The adjustment is the content.

Common Traps

A few habits, all reasonable, slow learning in clinical settings.

Waiting for certainty before contributing keeps unfinished thinking hidden, and unfinished thinking is exactly what a supervisor can help with. Certainty arrives far less often than the wait assumes.

Studying mainly to avoid being wrong on rounds aims at the wrong target. Clinical reasoning develops through encounters with uncertainty, so protecting yourself from error mostly removes you from the work that builds it.

Reading the discomfort of public learning as evidence of falling behind mistakes the format for a failing. Everyone learning in view feels exposed. The exposure is the arrangement, not a verdict.

Recap

What to hold onto when learning happens in front of people:

- In clinical training, knowledge develops in view instead of in private, which is a change in conditions, not a drop in ability.
- Questions on rounds usually surface reasoning so it can be taught, more than they test recall.
- Offering a tentative, partial answer opens the discussion that teaches, and silence closes it.
- New responsibility feels awkward because it arrives ahead of comfort, which is the shape of learning.
- You become more capable by participating before you feel ready.

Before You Move On

This chapter looked at how learning changes when it moves into public view, and why participating before you feel ready is how clinical reasoning develops.

Learning in the clinical years happens not only in front of people but inside institutions, each with its own expectations, feedback habits, and culture. The next chapter widens the frame to those systems, and to how much of what feels like a personal shortcoming is shaped by the environment a student is training in.

References

Benner, P. (1984). *From novice to expert: Excellence and power in clinical nursing practice.* Addison-Wesley.

Irby, D. M. (1995). Teaching and learning in ambulatory care settings: A thematic review of the literature. *Academic Medicine, 70*(10), 898–931.

CHAPTER SEVENTEEN

Students Learn Inside Systems

Key Question

How much of a hard rotation is you, and how much is the environment?

Core Idea

Curriculum, culture, and inconsistent feedback shape experience, so not every difficulty is a personal shortcoming.

Example Scenario

Sofia begins her third clinical rotation determined to do better.

She arrives early, stays late, reads about her patients, and actively seeks feedback. The effort is real, and she is genuinely committed to improving. Yet by the middle of the rotation, she feels increasingly discouraged.

The trouble is not a lack of effort. It is that expectations seem to change depending on who is evaluating her. Feedback from one supervisor conflicts with feedback from another. Some days she receives detailed guidance. Other days she receives almost none.

As the weeks pass, Sofia begins searching for explanations. The easiest explanation is personal. She assumes she is not adapting well enough, not learning quickly enough, or not meeting expectations consistently enough.

How well Sofia adapts is not something one rotation can measure. What she struggles to see is that part of her experience reflects the environment around her. Inconsistent feedback and shifting expectations are partly features of that environment, not signs that she is failing to adjust.

Why Individual Explanations Feel Natural

Students spend years receiving messages about personal responsibility: work harder, study smarter, manage your time, improve your habits.

These messages are not wrong. Individual choices influence learning, performance, and development. Students have real agency, and personal responsibility remains important throughout training.

The challenge emerges when individual explanations become the only explanations available.

When something goes poorly, students often look inward first. They search for flaws in effort, discipline, intelligence, or resilience. Sometimes those factors contribute to the problem. Sometimes they do not.

A student can work hard inside a poorly designed system. A student can use effective study strategies while receiving inconsistent feedback. A student can be performing adequately while training in an environment that increases stress and uncertainty.

When individual explanations dominate every interpretation, important parts of the situation become invisible.

Learning Never Happens in Isolation

Every learning environment contains structures that shape behavior.

Curricula determine what is taught and when. Assessment systems influence what students prioritize. Institutional culture influences what students believe is acceptable to discuss. Supervisors influence how feedback is delivered and interpreted.

These factors operate in the background of daily experience. Because they are always present, students often stop noticing them.

Yet these structures influence learning in meaningful ways. Students respond to incentives, expectations, and norms, not to information alone (O'Brien, Poncelet, & Hansen, 2010). The environment helps determine what receives attention and what is ignored.

This matters because students sometimes blame themselves for outcomes that are partly shaped by conditions around them.

Recognizing those conditions does not eliminate responsibility. It creates a more complete understanding of what is happening.

The Hidden Curriculum

Medical education includes more than formal instruction.

Students learn from lectures, readings, and clinical experiences. They also learn from observing how people behave, what gets rewarded, and what receives attention.

Researchers often describe this process as the hidden curriculum, the set of lessons communicated indirectly through culture and behavior instead of official teaching (Hafferty, 1998).

Students may hear that asking questions is encouraged while observing that uncertainty is sometimes punished. They may hear that well-being matters while observing that exhaustion is often admired. They may hear that learning is the priority while observing that performance receives most of the attention.

These contradictions can create confusion because students receive two sets of messages at the same time.

Understanding this dynamic helps explain why some experiences feel difficult to interpret. Students are responding to implicit expectations as much as explicit ones.

Why Feedback Feels Different Across Environments

Feedback plays a central role in learning.

Students rely on feedback to identify strengths, recognize weaknesses, and guide future improvement. Ideally, feedback provides information that supports growth.

In practice, feedback varies considerably.

Some supervisors provide clear, specific guidance you can actually use. Others offer vague comments that leave students uncertain about what should change. Some learning environments encourage regular feedback conversations, while others provide feedback only at major evaluation points.

Students often interpret differences in feedback quality as evidence about themselves.

A student receiving limited guidance may assume they are performing poorly. A student receiving inconsistent feedback may assume they are failing to understand expectations.

Sometimes the issue is not the student at all. It is the feedback system itself.

Understanding this distinction helps prevent students from drawing conclusions that the available information cannot support.

When Culture Shapes Interpretation

Students do not simply respond to events. They respond to the meaning attached to those events.

Culture plays an important role in shaping that meaning.

In some environments, mistakes are viewed primarily as opportunities for learning. In others, mistakes are interpreted as indicators of competence. In some environments, uncertainty is treated as a normal part of development. In others, uncertainty becomes something students try to hide.

These cultural differences influence how students experience the same event.

A missed question may feel like useful feedback in one setting and evidence of inadequacy in another. A request for help may feel responsible in one environment and risky in another.

The event remains the same. The interpretation changes because the surrounding culture changes.

The Danger of Personalizing System Problems

Students often carry responsibility for problems that extend beyond the individual.

A curriculum may be disorganized. Expectations may be unclear. Feedback may be inconsistent. Clinical responsibilities may conflict with learning needs.

These issues can create genuine difficulties.

The challenge is that students frequently interpret these difficulties as personal shortcomings. They assume that if they were more capable, more resilient, or better organized, the problem would disappear.

This interpretation creates unnecessary self-blame because it treats systemic issues as individual failures.

Recognizing the role of systems does not make students powerless. It means the source of a problem should be identified accurately before solutions are chosen.

A problem created by unclear expectations requires a different response than a problem created by inadequate preparation.

Maintaining Agency Without Taking All the Blame

Discussions about systems sometimes create concern that personal responsibility will disappear.

The opposite is usually true.

Accurate understanding allows students to direct effort where it can have the greatest impact. When students identify the actual source of a challenge, they can make more informed decisions about how to respond.

Agency becomes stronger when explanations become more accurate.

Students control some factors and do not control others. Productive adaptation requires distinguishing between the two. It often helps to ask what aspects of a situation can be influenced, what aspects fall outside one's control, what support or resources are available, which expectations are clear and which remain unclear, and what information is still missing. These questions focus attention on decisions you can actually make, instead of generalized frustration.

Deciding Where Your Effort Can Actually Land

The useful question is rarely whether a difficulty is entirely personal or entirely systemic, since most are some of both. Many learning problems do involve study habits, preparation, or skill, and those deserve real attention. The goal is to understand the interaction between the student and the environment, because learning happens at that intersection, and understanding both sides is what makes a response effective.

It helps to be honest about what the hidden curriculum actually rewards. Students hear that questions are welcome and watch uncertainty get punished. They hear that well-being matters and watch exhaustion get admired. When the stated message and the rewarded behavior diverge, the rewarded behavior is the real lesson, and reading inconsistent feedback as a verdict on yourself misses how much of it belongs to the system, not to you.

A couple of phrasings help when a standard is unclear: *Can you tell me specifically what a strong version of this would look like?* or, when feedback conflicts, *Dr. ___ suggested one approach and you're suggesting another. How should I prioritize between them?*

Try This Today

What to do: Think about a current challenge in your training. Write down your initial explanation for the problem. Then list factors that may exist at three levels: individual factors, interpersonal factors, and system factors.

What you may notice: Problems that initially seemed entirely personal often involve multiple contributing influences. The exercise does not eliminate responsibility, but it frequently creates a more complete picture.

Why it matters: Solutions become more effective when they match the actual sources of difficulty.

Options Menu

When a difficulty is partly the environment, these help separate what you can act on from what you cannot. If helpful:

- **Sort the problem into levels.** Name what is individual, what is interpersonal, and what is systemic before deciding what to fix.
- **Locate control.** Split what you can influence from what you cannot, and put effort into the first. It means accepting the second, and it sends energy where it can matter.

- **Ask for the standard explicitly.** When feedback is vague, request the specific expectation instead of inferring it. It feels exposing, and it turns a guessing game into information.

- **Find the second reading.** When feedback conflicts, ask which to prioritize instead of trying to satisfy both at once. It surfaces a contradiction that was never yours to resolve alone.

Common Traps

A few habits turn a system problem into a personal one.

Looking inward first feels like agency, *if I am the problem, I can fix it*, but reading every difficulty as a personal shortcoming hides the parts shaped by curriculum, culture, and inconsistent supervision, so they go unaddressed.

Reading limited or conflicting feedback as a final judgment draws a conclusion the information cannot support. The variation is often in the feedback system, not in you.

Personalizing a system problem keeps faith that more effort or resilience would dissolve it. A difficulty created by unclear expectations is not solved by trying harder inside the same fog.

Recap

What to hold onto when a rotation keeps feeling like your fault:

- **Learning happens inside systems**, and expectations, culture, and feedback shape what it feels like.

- **The hidden curriculum teaches through what gets rewarded,** not what gets stated.

- **Inconsistent feedback is often a property of the system,** not a verdict on you.

- **Naming the system's share does not cost you agency.** Accurate explanations make agency more effective.

- **Most situations are part individual and part environmental,** so the task is the interaction, not the blame.

Before You Move On

The previous chapter looked at learning in public. This one widened the frame to the systems that surround it: curriculum, culture, feedback, and the lessons taught indirectly by what gets rewarded. Much of what feels like a personal shortcoming is shaped by those conditions.

Conditions also operate at a much smaller scale, down to the single task a student cannot seem to begin. The next chapter examines avoidance, and why the inability to start is more often a response to how a task feels than a failure of character.

References

Hafferty, F. W. (1998). Beyond curriculum reform: Confronting medicine's hidden curriculum. *Academic Medicine, 73*(4), 403–407.

O'Brien, B. C., Poncelet, A. N., & Hansen, L. (2010). Students' workplace learning in two clerkships: A qualitative study. *Medical Education, 44*(6), 557–566.

C H A P T E R   E I G H T E E N

Avoidance Is Usually Trying to Solve a Problem

Key Question

Why can you know exactly what to do and still not start?

Core Idea

Avoidance is usually an attempt to manage discomfort, so the way through is to lower the cost of starting.

Example Scenario

Arjun knows exactly what he needs to do.

The exam is approaching, the material is unfinished, and the study plan is sitting open on his desk. He has already decided where to start. The resources are ready, the schedule is clear, and the next step is obvious.

An hour later, he is still not studying.

He has answered messages, reorganized his desk, checked his email, and read articles that have nothing to do with the exam. Throughout the entire hour, he remains aware of what he should be doing. The awareness makes the experience even more frustrating because he cannot explain why he is not starting.

A stalled hour reveals little about Arjun's discipline. The knowing is fully intact, since he can see exactly what to do, and that is the clue that *try harder* misreads what is happening here.

Why Avoidance Is So Easy to Misunderstand

Avoidance creates a confusing experience because students usually know what they should be doing. The problem is rarely a lack of information. Most students can identify the assignment, the exam, or the topic that requires attention.

This creates an important difference between knowing and doing. Students often assume that once a decision has been made, action should naturally follow. When action does not follow, they begin searching for explanations, and procrastination of this kind has less to do with poor time management than with the difficulty of self-regulation under emotional load (Steel, 2007).

The explanation that appears first is often personal. Students conclude that they are *lazy*, unmotivated, irresponsible, or insufficiently committed. These explanations feel convincing because they seem to match the behavior being observed.

The difficulty is that behavior alone does not explain why the behavior occurred. Two students can appear equally avoidant while responding to very different problems. Understanding avoidance requires looking beyond the visible behavior and examining the conditions that make action difficult.

Avoidance Often Reduces Distress

One reason avoidance persists is that it works, at least temporarily.

A difficult task often produces uncomfortable emotions. Students may feel overwhelmed, uncertain, intimidated, frustrated, or afraid of performing poorly. Beginning the task requires moving toward those feelings.

Avoidance provides a short-term alternative. By postponing the task, students also postpone the discomfort associated with it. The relief may last only a few minutes or a few hours, but it is often enough to reinforce the behavior. Avoidance, in this sense, prioritizes how a student feels right now over what the future self will need (Sirois & Pychyl, 2013).

Researchers Timothy Pychyl and Fuschia Sirois have described procrastination as closely connected to emotion regulation. From this perspective, avoidance is often more than a time-management problem. It is often an attempt to manage difficult emotional experiences (Pychyl & Sirois, 2016).

This interpretation does not make avoidance helpful. It makes avoidance easier to understand. The behavior is often trying to solve a problem, even when it creates larger problems later.

The Role of Overwhelm

Avoidance frequently appears when tasks become difficult to enter.

Chapter One described how cognitive load can make studying harder to start. Large, vague, and poorly defined tasks require substantial mental effort before meaningful work can begin.

Students often experience this as overwhelm. The amount of work feels larger than the capacity available to manage it. The task has too many components, too many decisions, or too many possible starting points.

In these situations, avoidance may have less to do with motivation than with task design. The student is facing a problem that lacks a clear entry point.

This distinction matters because the solution changes. If the problem is interpreted as laziness, the response is usually more pressure. If the problem is task overload, the response may involve reducing complexity and clarifying the next action.

The second response often produces better results because it addresses the mechanism creating the resistance.

The Role of Uncertainty

Students often assume that difficult tasks are avoided because they are unpleasant.

Sometimes tasks are avoided because they are uncertain.

Uncertainty creates its own form of discomfort. A student may not know whether they understand the material, whether their study method is working, or whether the effort invested will produce the desired outcome. Beginning the task requires confronting that uncertainty directly.

Practice questions provide a useful example. Many students know that practice questions are valuable. They also know that questions can expose weaknesses, reveal gaps in knowledge, and challenge assumptions about preparedness.

The task becomes emotionally complicated because it offers information the student wants and fears at the same time.

Avoidance can emerge when uncertainty becomes difficult to tolerate. The issue is not that the student does not care. It is that caring makes the uncertainty matter.

The Role of Self-Protection

Some forms of avoidance function as protection.

Students occasionally delay tasks because beginning would require confronting the possibility of performing poorly. As long as the task remains unfinished, the outcome remains unknown.

This does not mean students consciously decide to avoid disappointment. Most avoidance operates much more automatically than that.

The important point is that performance carries meaning. Students who tie academic outcomes closely to identity may experience greater emotional risk when approaching evaluative tasks. A question block, practice exam, or challenging assignment can begin to feel like more than an academic exercise.

When the task becomes a test of worth, avoidance often becomes more likely.

The student is no longer approaching a learning activity. They are approaching something that feels personally consequential.

Why More Pressure Often Fails

Students frequently respond to avoidance by increasing self-criticism.

They call themselves *lazy*, tell themselves to *stop making excuses*, and attempt to generate motivation through pressure. Sometimes this works temporarily. More often, it creates additional distress.

The problem is that pressure does not reliably solve the issues that commonly produce avoidance. It does not reduce cognitive load, clarify uncertainty, or simplify task entry. In some cases, it increases the emotional burden already attached to the work.

This is one reason students sometimes become trapped in a cycle of avoidance and self-criticism. Avoidance creates guilt. Guilt increases emotional discomfort. Increased discomfort makes the task harder to approach. The result is more avoidance.

Understanding the cycle does not excuse it. It helps explain why pressure alone often fails to interrupt it.

There is a counterintuitive way out of the loop. In one study, students who forgave themselves for procrastinating before an exam went on to procrastinate less before the next one (Wohl et al., 2010). Releasing the self-blame reduced the negative feeling attached to the task, which made it easier to approach the next time. Self-forgiveness, in other words, lowers the barrier to starting again.

Making the Task Easier to Enter

Many effective responses to avoidance focus on task design instead of motivation. Reducing the size of the task lowers the cost of entry, clarifying the first action removes decisions, and separating planning from execution reduces the thinking required before work begins.

Smaller tasks can seem less serious, but a large task that never begins produces little learning, while a small one that begins immediately often creates momentum the larger plan never reaches. The goal is not to lower standards. It is to reduce the barrier between intention and action.

The Difference Between Resistance and Refusal

Students often interpret any difficulty starting as evidence that they do not want to do the work.

A cleaner distinction separates resistance from refusal.

Refusal means choosing not to engage. Resistance means wanting to engage while encountering barriers that make engagement difficult.

Many students experiencing avoidance are actually experiencing resistance. They care deeply about the outcome. They understand the importance of the task. They fully intend to begin.

The conflict comes from the presence of competing forces. Part of the student wants to move toward the task. Another part wants to move away from the discomfort associated with it.

Recognizing this distinction changes the conversation. The problem becomes identifying the barrier instead of questioning the student's commitment.

Try This Today

What to do: Choose one study task you have been avoiding. Instead of focusing on completing the entire task, identify the smallest meaningful action that would move it forward. Commit to that action only.

What you may notice: The resistance often decreases once the task becomes concrete and limited. The emotional burden attached to beginning may feel smaller than expected.

Why it matters: Avoidance often grows around large, ambiguous tasks. Reducing the entry cost makes action easier without lowering the importance of the work.

Avoidance wins in the moment of deciding, so decide in advance. Pair the predictable stall with a small, pre-set action, and the response is settled before the discomfort arrives. *If I notice I have been avoiding the question bank, then I open it and do two questions, only two. If a task feels too big to start, then I name the smallest first action and do that.* The point is to remove the in-the-moment choice, which is where avoidance lives.

Options Menu

Most of what helps with avoidance lowers the cost of starting instead of raising the pressure. If helpful:

- **Shrink to the smallest meaningful action.** Reduce the task until a clear first step appears. The step can look trivial, and a small task that begins beats a large one that does not.

- **Forgive the last stall.** Letting go of self-blame from the last avoidance has been shown to make the next start easier (Wohl et al.,

2010). It feels like letting yourself off the hook, and it removes the guilt that was fueling the avoidance.

- **Name the feeling you're avoiding.** Overwhelm, uncertainty, or fear of a poor result each point to a different fix. It takes a moment of honesty, and it tells you which problem avoidance is solving.
- **Separate planning from doing.** Decide the first step in advance so beginning requires no further decision. A little setup removes the deliberation avoidance feeds on.
- **Build an If/Then for the recurring stall.** Pre-decide the response to the avoidance you can already predict.

Common Traps

A few responses to avoidance deepen the cycle they are meant to break.

Reading avoidance as a discipline failure fits the visible behavior while missing the mechanism. The same stall can come from overwhelm, uncertainty, or self-protection, and *try harder* addresses none of them.

Answering avoidance with self-criticism assumes pressure produces action. More often it adds guilt, guilt adds discomfort, and discomfort makes the task harder to approach, the cycle the chapter describes.

Refusing small tasks as not serious enough protects a standard and guarantees the large task keeps not starting. Momentum comes from entry, not from the size of the plan.

Recap

What to hold onto when you cannot seem to start:

- **Avoidance is usually solving a problem (managing overwhelm**, uncertainty, or risk), not revealing a flaw.
- **The mechanism is hidden while the behavior is visible,** which is why it reads as character.
- Pressure rarely fixes what produces avoidance and often deepens the cycle.
- **Resistance (wanting to start**, blocked) and refusal (choosing not to) are different, and most stalls are resistance.
- **Lower the cost of entry.** The smallest real action beats the largest unstarted plan.

Before You Move On

The previous chapter examined the systems students learn inside. This chapter narrowed to a single stalled task and looked at avoidance as a response to how the work feels, not a failure of character.

Avoidance shapes what students do. A related difficulty shapes how they feel about themselves while doing it. Many students move through training carrying a persistent sense that they are falling behind or underperforming, even when the evidence runs the other way. The next chapter examines self-doubt, why it becomes so common in high-achieving environments, and how to evaluate your ability without turning uncertainty into a permanent conclusion.

References

Pychyl, T. A., & Sirois, F. M. (2016). Procrastination, emotion regulation, and well-being. In F. M. Sirois & T. A. Pychyl (Eds.), *Procrastination, health, and well-being* (pp. 163–188). Academic Press.

Sirois, F. M., & Pychyl, T. A. (2013). Procrastination and the priority of short-term mood regulation: Consequences for future self. *Social and Personality Psychology Compass, 7*(2), 115–127.

Steel, P. (2007). The nature of procrastination: A meta-analytic and theoretical review of quintessential self-regulatory failure. *Psychological Bulletin, 133*(1), 65–94.

Wohl, M. J. A., Pychyl, T. A., & Bennett, S. H. (2010). I forgive myself, now I can study: How self-forgiveness for procrastinating can reduce future procrastination. *Personality and Individual Differences, 48*(7), 803–808.

Part Five

When Effort Isn't Enough

The earlier parts of this book treated studying as a system: load, access, strategy, the emotions that draw on that same capacity, the recovery that sets its ceiling, and the environments it happens inside. Understanding those conditions changes what a student can do.

It does not make training easy. Even with sound methods and an accurate read on the system, medical education keeps producing experiences that effort alone does not resolve. Self-doubt persists after good results. Progress refuses to move in a straight line. Real failure arrives, carrying more weight than any single result should. Each of these is part of what a learning system has to withstand.

This final part takes up those experiences directly. Chapter Nineteen examines self-doubt, and why it so often outlasts the evidence. Chapter Twenty looks at the uneven shape of progress, and why a plateau or a dip is rarely what it feels like. Chapter Twenty-One turns to failure, and how a result can become information rather than a verdict. Chapter Twenty-Two draws the threads together into a learning system built to keep working when conditions do not cooperate.

The aim is a way of learning that keeps working when training is at its hardest.

CHAPTER NINETEEN

Self-Doubt Is Not Always Diagnostic

Key Question

When is self-doubt accurate information, and when is it just a feeling?

Core Idea

Doubt reports on your experience, and in medicine it can persist regardless of real competence.

Example Scenario

Emma receives her exam score and immediately begins calculating what it means.

The score is not disastrous. In fact, it is close to the class average. Objectively, there is little evidence that anything is seriously wrong. Yet by the end of the day, Emma is questioning her abilities, replaying mistakes, and wondering whether everyone else is adapting more successfully than she is.

The score itself occupies only a small part of her attention. Most of her energy is directed toward interpreting what the score seems to reveal about her future. She is no longer evaluating a performance. She is evaluating herself.

A score near the class average tells Emma little about her future. What stands out is where her attention went: off the performance and onto a verdict about herself.

Why Self-Doubt Feels So Convincing

Self-doubt is persuasive because it usually presents itself as caution, not distortion.

Students rarely think, *I am being unfair to myself.* Instead, they think they are being realistic. They assume that questioning their abilities protects them from complacency, overconfidence, or future disappointment.

This interpretation makes self-doubt difficult to challenge. The doubts often appear responsible and thoughtful. They seem like signs of humility, not signs of distress.

The problem is that self-doubt frequently operates without requiring much evidence. A difficult week can trigger it. A disappointing exam can trigger it. Sometimes comparison, uncertainty, or exhaustion can trigger it.

Once activated, self-doubt often begins collecting information that supports its conclusions while ignoring information that challenges them.

Why Competence Does Not Eliminate Doubt

Students often assume that confidence arrives naturally with competence (Bandura, 1997).

The expectation seems reasonable. If uncertainty comes from not knowing enough, then acquiring knowledge should solve the problem. If doubt comes from inexperience, then experience should eliminate it.

Medical education frequently challenges this assumption. Students gain knowledge while simultaneously becoming more aware of what they do not know. As understanding grows, awareness of complexity often grows as well. Questions become more sophisticated, responsibilities become greater, and uncertainty becomes harder to avoid.

As a result, competence and self-doubt can coexist. A student may perform well while still feeling uncertain. The experience of feeling like a fraud despite real accomplishment is common enough among high achievers to have its own name in the research literature (Clance & Imes, 1978). Another student may receive positive evaluations while continuing to question whether they belong. Seen against a developmental arc like the one described in Chapter Sixteen, persistent uncertainty reads as the texture of still being on the path. The presence of self-doubt does not automatically indicate the absence of ability.

The Problem With Using Feelings as Evidence

Students often treat feelings as if they are measurements.

Feeling behind becomes evidence of being behind. Feeling unprepared becomes evidence of being unprepared. Feeling inadequate becomes evidence of inadequacy.

The difficulty is that feelings provide information about experience, not necessarily about reality.

Anxiety can create feelings of danger in situations that are manageable. Comparison can create feelings of inferiority in situations where meaningful progress is occurring. Self-doubt can create feelings of incompetence even when performance suggests otherwise.

This does not mean feelings should be ignored. They matter because they influence behavior, attention, and decision-making.

The point is more specific. Feelings should be considered as data, not treated as proof.

Why Medical Training Creates Persistent Uncertainty

Many professions allow people to develop a stable sense of competence relatively quickly.

Medical education works differently.

Students spend years operating near the edge of their knowledge. New information arrives continuously. Responsibilities expand faster than confidence. Every stage of training introduces tasks that once seemed impossible.

The result is an environment where uncertainty remains normal even as competence increases.

This observation matters because students often interpret uncertainty as evidence that they are not progressing. In reality, uncertainty may be an unavoidable consequence of learning increasingly complex material.

A student can be improving substantially while continuing to feel unsure. The feeling alone cannot determine which explanation is correct.

When Self-Doubt Becomes Self-Protection

Some forms of self-doubt function as protection.

Students sometimes believe that maintaining a critical view of themselves will keep them motivated. They worry that confidence will lead to complacency, mistakes, or decreased effort.

The intention makes sense. Medicine requires seriousness, attention to detail, and ongoing learning.

The problem is that excessive self-doubt often creates costs that outweigh its benefits. It can increase anxiety, reduce willingness to attempt difficult tasks, and make setbacks feel more threatening than they need to be.

Students do not need constant self-criticism to remain committed to improvement. Most medical students already care deeply about performing well.

The challenge is learning how to pursue growth without turning every weakness into evidence of inadequacy.

Separating Growth From Judgment

Improvement requires recognizing weaknesses.

Students need feedback. They need accurate assessments of performance. They need opportunities to identify gaps and address them.

None of these tasks require harsh self-judgment. Treating yourself with the same steadiness you would offer a struggling colleague tends to support improvement instead of undermining it (Neff, 2011).

Growth and judgment often become intertwined because students assume that criticism produces improvement. Sometimes criticism simply produces distress.

A steadier approach begins with description instead of evaluation. Instead of deciding what a weakness means about the student, attention remains focused on what the weakness actually is.

The question changes from *What does this say about me?* to *What skill needs development?*

This shift preserves accountability while reducing unnecessary conclusions about identity.

Evidence Matters More Than Impressions

Calibration appeared earlier in the book because evidence is the counterbalance to self-doubt. A student who relies on impressions alone is at the mercy of whichever feeling is loudest, so a difficult day starts to define a semester and a disappointing result starts to define an identity.

Performance trends, practice questions, feedback from trusted supervisors, and completed work all supply evidence. It does not eliminate uncertainty, but it is a steadier foundation than a passing emotional state, and the goal is not complete confidence. It is conclusions supported by more than a feeling.

What You Would Conclude About Someone Else

The same consistency test from Chapter Twelve applies here. A classmate who performs near the average after a hard block, or who voices uncertainty on a rotation, usually receives an understanding read, while the identical performance in oneself becomes evidence of falling short. Asking what you would conclude about another capable student in the same position holds one standard instead of two, and it tends to produce a more accurate conclusion than self-judgment does.

Try This Today

What to do: When self-doubt becomes particularly strong, write down the specific conclusion you are reaching. Then create two columns. In the first column, list the evidence supporting that conclusion. In the second column, list the evidence challenging it.

What you may notice: The evidence is often more mixed than the initial conclusion suggested. Strong feelings frequently create the impression that the case is already settled.

Why it matters: Self-doubt often feels persuasive because it presents conclusions without requiring a careful review of the evidence. The exercise slows that process down and creates room for a more balanced interpretation.

Options Menu

The shift turns one strong feeling into evidence, and these are other ways to keep self-doubt from settling into a conclusion. If helpful:

- **Build the evidence list.** Set the feeling beside what supports and challenges it. It reopens a case the feeling had closed.

- **Describe the weakness instead of judging it.** Move from *what does this mean about me?* to *what specifically needs work?* It is less dramatic than a verdict, and it keeps accountability without the distress.

- **Weigh trends over impressions.** Place the prominent feeling next to performance over time. It is slower than the feeling, and it is the more reliable evidence.

- **Apply the consistency test.** Ask what you would conclude about a capable classmate in the same position (see Chapter Twelve).

Common Traps

Self-doubt is convincing precisely because it does not look like distortion.

Treating self-doubt as realism feels like humility, which is exactly why it goes unchallenged while it collects evidence for its own conclusions and overlooks the rest.

Using feelings as measurements turns *I feel behind* into *I am behind.* Feelings report on experience, and in a field built on working near the edge of your knowledge, the feeling of not-enough is nearly constant regardless of performance.

Keeping a harsh view of yourself to stay motivated assumes criticism drives improvement. Growth needs accurate feedback. The condemnation mostly adds cost.

Recap

What to hold onto when doubt outlasts the evidence:

- **Self-doubt presents as caution**, which is why it rarely gets questioned.
- **Competence and doubt coexist,** and in medicine, awareness of complexity grows as fast as knowledge.
- **Feelings are data about experience**, not proof about reality.
- Description (***what skill needs work?***) **keeps accountability.** Judgment (*what does this say about me?*) mostly produces distress.
- Evidence over time is a steadier foundation than whichever feeling is loudest today.

Before You Move On

The previous chapter looked at avoidance. This chapter examined self-doubt, and how uncertainty can harden into a conclusion about ability even when the evidence is thin.

Self-doubt feeds on a particular misreading of progress: the assumption that learning should be steadily visible, so that any dip means something has gone wrong. The next chapter takes up the shape of progress itself, and why improvement is almost never the straight line students expect.

References

Bandura, A. (1997). *Self-efficacy: The exercise of control.* Freeman.

Clance, P. R., & Imes, S. A. (1978). The imposter phenomenon in high achieving women: Dynamics and therapeutic intervention. *Psychotherapy: Theory, Research & Practice, 15*(3), 241–247.

Neff, K. D. (2011). *Self-compassion: The proven power of being kind to yourself.* William Morrow.

CHAPTER TWENTY

Progress Is Usually Uneven

Key Question

Why does real progress often look like a plateau or a dip?

Core Idea

Learning develops below the surface of performance, so trends carry more information than any single moment.

Example Scenario

Jamal has been doing everything he can think of.

He is completing practice questions, reviewing missed concepts, and following a study schedule that feels more organized than anything he has used before. For several weeks, the work seems to be paying off. Scores improve, retrieval becomes easier, and studying feels more manageable.

Then something changes.

A question set goes poorly. Concepts that seemed solid suddenly feel uncertain. A practice exam score drops below expectations. Within a few days, Jamal begins wondering whether all of the recent effort has stopped working.

After several good weeks, one dip is no sign the work stopped working. The point is the expectation it violates: that real learning should rise in a straight line.

The experience feels alarming because students often expect improvement to follow a predictable pattern. If learning is occurring, performance should steadily improve. If performance declines, learning must no longer be occurring.

Learning rarely works that way.

Many students enter medical school with an implicit belief that progress should be visible, consistent, and easy to recognize. When improvement becomes uneven, they often interpret normal variability as evidence that something is wrong.

This chapter examines why progress is often irregular, why setbacks frequently occur during periods of genuine development, and why isolated moments provide less information than students often assume.

Why We Expect Progress to Be Linear

Most students have spent years using grades and scores as indicators of progress.

The structure encourages a simple expectation. More effort should produce better performance. Better performance should indicate improvement. The relationship appears straightforward.

This expectation becomes harder to maintain in medical school because learning tasks become more complex. Students are doing more than memorizing information. They are building knowledge structures, developing clinical reasoning, learning to tolerate uncertainty, and integrating information across disciplines.

These forms of development do not always produce immediate improvements in performance. Sometimes growth becomes visible only after a delay.

The difficulty is that students continue evaluating themselves using expectations developed in environments where progress was easier to observe.

When improvement becomes less visible, students often assume it has stopped.

Learning Often Looks Messier Than It Feels

Students frequently imagine learning as a steady upward trajectory.

The reality is usually more complicated. Progress often includes periods of improvement, plateaus, temporary declines, and unexpected jumps forward.

Part of this variability reflects the complexity of learning itself. As students encounter more difficult material, performance may temporarily worsen even while understanding deepens. New information can disrupt existing patterns before stronger ones emerge.

The process can feel discouraging because performance is visible while underlying development is not (Bjork & Bjork, 2011).

A student may experience a temporary decline and conclude that learning has failed. In reality, the decline may be occurring during a period of substantial adaptation.

Not every setback represents growth. The point is narrower: setbacks alone cannot determine whether growth is occurring.

The Problem With Small Samples

Students often draw large conclusions from small amounts of information.

A difficult day becomes evidence of a difficult month. A disappointing exam becomes evidence of a disappointing year. A poor question block becomes evidence that a study strategy is failing.

These interpretations are understandable because negative experiences naturally attract attention. The emotional impact of a setback often exceeds its informational value.

One poor performance provides limited evidence about a larger trend. Performance fluctuates for many reasons, including fatigue, stress, question difficulty, attention, and random variation.

Students usually understand this principle when evaluating scientific data. They are less likely to apply the same principle when evaluating themselves.

A single observation rarely provides enough information to support a broad conclusion.

Why Plateaus Feel So Discouraging

Plateaus create a unique challenge because they often feel like stagnation.

Students continue investing effort while receiving little visible evidence of improvement. Retrieval remains difficult. Scores remain relatively stable. The work continues, but progress appears absent.

The experience can be frustrating because effort and results no longer seem connected. Students begin questioning their methods, their abilities, or their future prospects.

Plateaus often occur because development is taking place below the level of immediate performance. Knowledge structures may be becoming more organized. Connections may be strengthening. Skills may be becoming more efficient. This fits the developmental picture from Chapter Sixteen: movement toward expertise comes through stages and through experience in real situations, and it rarely advances at a constant rate.

These changes are difficult to observe directly.

The challenge is that students evaluate progress using measures that may lag behind the underlying learning process.

Temporary Setbacks Are Not Permanent Trends

Medical students are often surrounded by high-stakes evaluations. This environment encourages constant monitoring of performance. Every score, ranking, and assessment can begin to feel highly significant.

The result is that temporary setbacks often receive more weight than they deserve.

A lower score feels like a trend. A difficult week feels like a trajectory. Students begin projecting current struggles into the future.

Set the two side by side: moments spike and carry the feeling, while the slower trend beneath them carries the information.

The problem is that performance snapshots do not reliably predict long-term outcomes.

Most students who complete medical training can identify periods when progress felt slow, uncertain, or invisible. Those periods often looked much more meaningful while they were happening than they did in retrospect.

This observation is not meant to minimize setbacks. It is meant to place them in context.

Why High Achievers Struggle With Variability

Many medical students are accustomed to consistent success.

Earlier educational experiences often reinforced the belief that effort should produce predictable results (Dweck, 2006). Variability existed, but it was usually limited enough that overall progress felt stable.

Medical school introduces more uncertainty.

The material is more complex. The expectations are less familiar. The evaluations are often more challenging. Under these conditions, performance becomes more variable.

Students who are unaccustomed to variability may interpret it as evidence of decline.

A more accurate interpretation is that variability becomes normal as tasks become more demanding.

The presence of fluctuation does not necessarily indicate the absence of growth.

Looking for Trends Instead of Moments

Individual events draw attention because they are emotionally vivid: a hard exam, a disappointing block, a frustrating session all stay with you. Learning is easier to read across longer stretches, by asking whether performance differs from a few months ago and whether this month's mistakes are the same ones or new ones. Trends generally carry better information than individual observations.

The Difference Between Slow and Stuck

Students often use the word "stuck" when progress feels slower than expected.

Sometimes students are genuinely stuck. A study strategy may be ineffective. A knowledge gap may require attention. Additional support may be needed.

More often, students are progressing more slowly than they would prefer.

The distinction matters because slow progress and absent progress are different situations.

When students confuse the two, they may abandon effective strategies prematurely. They may change approaches repeatedly, searching for evidence of immediate improvement.

Learning frequently requires more patience than students find comfortable.

The challenge is remaining engaged long enough for progress to become visible.

Try This Today

What to do: Take the setback that is worrying you and gather three or four more data points around it: recent scores, and the kinds of mistakes you are making now compared with a month ago. Look at the trend they form instead of the single moment.

What you may notice: A bad block rarely survives contact with the surrounding trend, and plateaus often sit on top of development that is not visible yet.

Why it matters: Performance lags learning, and one vivid moment carries more feeling than information. The reading that tells the truth is the pattern across weeks, not the worst recent point.

Decide in advance how you will read a dip, so a single bad day does not get to write the trend. *If one block goes badly, then I log it and wait for two more before changing anything. If progress feels stalled, then I compare this month's mistakes with last month's before concluding I am stuck.* Pre-deciding the interpretation keeps a vivid moment from becoming a verdict.

Options Menu

When progress is hard to read, these keep the reading accurate. If helpful:

- **Judge trends, not moments.** Gather several data points around a setback and read the pattern. A slower verdict, and a truer one.

- **Distinguish slow from stuck.** Ask whether progress is absent or merely slower than you would like before changing strategy. It takes patience, and it keeps you from abandoning a method mid-stride.

- **Track mistake-type over time.** Notice whether this month's errors differ from last month's. It is less satisfying than a score, and changing error patterns are evidence a score can hide.

Common Traps

A few expectations make ordinary progress hard to see.

Expecting progress to be linear carries forward a model from earlier schooling, where effort and results tracked closely. Medical-school learning develops below the surface of performance, so the old model reads normal dips as decline.

Drawing a trend from one performance answers the wish to know immediately where you stand. A single block is a small sample shaped by fatigue, difficulty, and chance, and rarely supports the conclusion the feeling wants.

Reading a plateau as stagnation mistakes the lag between learning and visible performance for an absence of learning, which is exactly when students tend to abandon methods that were working.

Recap

What to hold onto when progress stalls or dips:

- Learning is uneven, and improvement, plateaus, dips, and jumps are the normal shape, not a malfunction.
- Performance lags learning, so development often becomes visible only after a delay.
- **One block is a small sample.** Trends carry the information, and moments carry the feeling.
- **Slow progress and absent progress are different**, and confusing them makes you quit working methods early.
- A plateau is often organization happening below the level you can yet measure.

Before You Move On

The previous chapter examined self-doubt. This chapter looked at the uneven shape of progress, and the pull to read a temporary setback as a permanent trend.

Progress that dips is one thing. Outright failure is another. A failed exam or a poor evaluation carries weight a plateau does not. The next chapter takes up failure directly, and how a result can become information rather than a verdict on who you are.

References

Bjork, E. L., & Bjork, R. A. (2011). Making things hard on yourself, but in a good way: Creating desirable difficulties to enhance learning. In M. A. Gernsbacher, R. W. Pew, L. M. Hough, & J. R. Pomerantz

(Eds.), *Psychology and the real world: Essays illustrating fundamental contributions to society* (pp. 56–64). Worth.

Dweck, C. S. (2006). *Mindset: The new psychology of success.* Random House.

CHAPTER TWENTY-ONE

Failure Is Data

Key Question

How do you respond to failure without turning it into a verdict?

Core Idea

A failure tells you what happened under specific conditions, and its value comes from making that specific.

Example Scenario

Alyssa fails an exam.

The result feels impossible to process at first. She reopens the score report several times, hoping she misunderstood something. For months she has been working hard, attending lectures, completing practice questions, and trying to stay on top of the workload. None of that effort seems visible in the result.

Within hours, a new question begins to dominate her thinking.

What does this mean about me?

The question feels natural because failure often arrives with emotional consequences that extend far beyond the event itself. A failed exam can threaten confidence, disrupt plans, and raise concerns about the future. Students rarely experience failure as a neutral piece of information.

A single failed exam is not a measure of who Alyssa is or what she can become. What stands out is how quickly the result recruited a much larger question about her.

A failure belongs inside a cycle: an attempt, an error, the feedback it produces, an adjustment, and the next attempt.

Why Failure Feels So Final

Most academic experiences provide some opportunity for recovery.

A missed question affects a score slightly. A disappointing assignment can often be balanced by future performance. Small mistakes are absorbed into larger patterns.

Failure feels different because it appears categorical.

The exam was passed or failed. The evaluation was satisfactory or unsatisfactory. The application was accepted or rejected. The outcome seems clear, which creates the impression that its meaning is equally clear.

Students often respond by treating the result as a comprehensive assessment of ability. A failed exam becomes evidence that they are not capable enough. A poor evaluation becomes evidence that they are not developing appropriately.

The emotional logic is understandable. The difficulty is that outcomes rarely explain themselves.

A result tells you what happened. It does not automatically tell you why.

Failure Answers Fewer Questions Than Students Think

When students experience failure, they often feel as though a large number of questions have suddenly been answered.

The score appears to reveal intelligence, preparedness, future success, and belonging all at once. The experience feels definitive because the result is visible and difficult to ignore.

In reality, failure usually answers a much narrower question.

A failed exam demonstrates that performance on a particular assessment did not meet a required standard under specific conditions. That information matters. It deserves careful attention.

What it does not reveal is equally important.

Failure does not automatically explain motivation, potential, worth, future competence, or long-term outcomes. Those conclusions often arrive quickly, but they extend beyond the available evidence.

The challenge is learning how to separate the result from the interpretations attached to it.

The Difference Between Outcome and Cause

Students often focus on outcomes because outcomes are obvious.

The exam score is visible. The evaluation is visible. The failed attempt is visible. Causes are usually more difficult to identify.

A failed outcome may emerge from many different factors. Knowledge gaps, ineffective study strategies, retrieval problems, fatigue, anxiety, poor calibration, inadequate preparation, health concerns, or environmental challenges can all contribute.

Different causes require different responses.

A student who failed because of weak retrieval needs a different plan than a student who failed because of severe exhaustion. A student struggling with cognitive overload requires a different intervention than a student struggling with ineffective study methods.

The usefulness of failure depends on understanding what produced it.

Without that analysis, students often respond to every failure in the same way: by working harder.

Additional effort sometimes helps. Sometimes it leaves the underlying problem unchanged.

Why High Achievers Often Struggle With Failure

Many medical students have relatively little experience with major academic failure.

Their previous educational experiences were often characterized by competence, achievement, and steady progress. Failure existed, but it was usually limited in scope and frequency.

As a result, failure can feel unfamiliar.

Students who have not developed frameworks for interpreting failure may experience it primarily as a threat. The event appears inconsistent with how they understand themselves.

This tension often creates urgency. Students want immediate explanations and immediate solutions. The discomfort of uncertainty can make careful analysis difficult.

Unfortunately, quick explanations are not always accurate explanations.

Failure becomes more useful when students can tolerate uncertainty long enough to investigate what actually happened.

Experts and Novices Use Failure Differently

One difference between developing learners and experts involves how mistakes are interpreted.

Novices often treat mistakes as evaluations. The mistake becomes evidence about ability, intelligence, or potential.

Experts are more likely to treat mistakes as information. Research on expert performance describes development as a process of using feedback from errors to target the next round of practice (Ericsson, 2004).

Experts are not immune to disappointment, and they take no special pleasure in failure. What differs is that their attention moves more quickly toward understanding the mechanisms involved. They ask what specifically went wrong, what conditions contributed, what skill requires improvement, what evidence supports the conclusion, and what should change next time.

These questions do not remove the emotional impact of failure. They help transform failure into something that can guide future action.

Failure Becomes Useful When It Becomes Specific

Students often describe failures in broad terms.

Statements such as "I failed" or "I am struggling" communicate emotional reality, but they provide limited guidance for improvement.

Specific descriptions are usually more useful.

A student may have struggled with retrieval, time management, question interpretation, anxiety, foundational understanding, or preparation strategy. Each possibility points toward a different response.

Specificity matters because solutions emerge from mechanisms, not labels.

The more accurately a student can describe the problem, the easier it becomes to identify a meaningful adjustment.

This process requires honesty, but it does not require self-condemnation.

Ask the Task, Not Yourself

The kind of feedback you seek changes what it can do for you.

Global questions, like *how did I do?* or *am I behind?*, invite an answer aimed at the self, and feedback aimed at the self tends to help least. A large review of feedback studies found that when feedback directs attention to the person instead of the task, it can leave performance unchanged or even lower it (Kluger & DeNisi, 1996). This is the judgment-versus-description distinction from earlier, arriving now from the outside.

Task-level questions do more work. *Was my differential ordered sensibly? Did I miss a step in the workup? Where did my reasoning turn?* These direct the response to something specific and changeable, which is where the next adjustment comes from (Hattie & Timperley, 2007). The more precise the question, the more usable the answer.

The move is the same one this chapter already makes with failure: replace the verdict with the mechanism. Applied to feedback, it means asking for information about the work, not a rating of the self.

The Danger of Global Conclusions

One of the most common responses to failure is overgeneralization.

A student fails one exam and begins questioning their entire future. A difficult rotation raises doubts about overall competence. One disappointing outcome expands into a broad conclusion about identity. Beliefs about whether ability is fixed or capable of developing shape how far that conclusion travels (Dweck, 2006).

The mind often moves in this direction because global explanations feel complete. They reduce uncertainty by providing a simple story. The difficulty is that broad conclusions are frequently supported by limited evidence.

A failed exam is meaningful. It deserves attention. It does not automatically justify conclusions about an entire career.

Students often benefit from asking whether the conclusion they are reaching extends beyond what the evidence can reasonably support.

This question creates space for more accurate interpretation.

Adaptation Requires Feedback

Failure becomes valuable when it produces useful feedback. The point of analysis is not to dwell on the mistake but to identify the adjustment that makes the next attempt more likely to succeed, and that adjustment depends on matching the response to the cause, as the rest of the book has argued.

Failure often becomes less overwhelming once it generates a concrete plan. The emotional weight may remain, but the uncertainty starts to lift, and a path forward becomes visible.

Try This Today

What to do: Think about a recent setback. Describe the event as specifically as possible, focusing on observable facts before attempting to explain what the event means. Then ask: What happened? What factors contributed? Which factors are most likely to matter? What evidence supports those conclusions? What specific change should occur next?

What you may notice: The initial explanation often becomes more nuanced. Broad conclusions frequently become narrower and easier to act on.

Why it matters: Failure becomes easier to learn from when it is analyzed before it is judged.

Regrouping Plan

After a significant setback, a short structured reset works better than either pushing harder or starting over. Three questions usually do it: what pattern actually appeared, beyond this one event; which condition most likely contributed (load, access, strategy, emotion, recovery, or systems); and what single change fits that condition next time. The adjustment is small on purpose, because small changes survive the disruption a failure creates. The fuller version, for rebuilding a whole study cycle, appears in Chapter Twenty-Two.

Options Menu

These turn a result into information. If helpful:

- **Run a failure review.** Lay out the facts before the meaning. It sits with the event longer than is comfortable, and it analyzes before it judges.

- **Make the failure specific.** Replace *I failed* with the mechanism: retrieval, timing, interpretation, foundations, anxiety. It takes honesty, and specificity is where the next move comes from.

- **Regroup with a single change.** Reset around one adjustment instead of overhauling everything. It is slower than resolving to try harder, and it matches the response to the cause.

- **Check the conclusion against the evidence.** Ask whether the conclusion you are reaching extends past what one result can support. It leaves some uncertainty intact, and it keeps one outcome from becoming a conclusion about a career.

Common Traps

A few responses to failure keep its information out of reach.

Treating a failure as a verdict assumes a clear outcome has a clear meaning. Pass or fail is categorical, but the result tells you what happened, not why, and the why is where every useful response lives.

Answering every failure by working harder reaches for the one lever that has always seemed available. Different causes (retrieval, exhaustion, calibration, conditions) need different responses, and effort aimed at the wrong one leaves it untouched.

Letting one result expand into a global conclusion supplies a complete story by closing the question early. Broad conclusions about ability or belonging tend to rest on a single data point that cannot carry them.

Recap

What to hold onto after a real setback:

- A failure tells you a specific performance missed a standard under specific conditions. That, and nothing more.
- **Result and cause are different.** The result is visible, and the cause needs analysis.
- **Failure becomes useful when it becomes specific: the mechanism**, not the label.
- **Different causes need different responses**, and *work harder* is not a universal fix.

- **Analyze before you judge.** One result rarely supports a conclusion about who you are.

Before You Move On

This chapter examined more substantial failures and how students can respond to them without turning them into judgments about identity.

Failure is difficult because it carries emotional weight. At the same time, failure often contains information that success does not provide. Mistakes reveal weaknesses, assumptions, and gaps that would otherwise remain hidden.

The challenge is learning how to use that information effectively.

The next chapter brings together many of the ideas from this book and focuses on building a sustainable learning system. Rather than treating studying as a collection of isolated techniques, we will examine how retrieval, recovery, calibration, feedback, and adaptation can work together over time.

References

Dweck, C. S. (2006). *Mindset: The new psychology of success.* Random House.

Ericsson, K. A. (2004). Deliberate practice and the acquisition and maintenance of expert performance in medicine and related domains. *Academic Medicine, 79*(10 Suppl), S70–S81.

Hattie, J., & Timperley, H. (2007). The power of feedback. *Review of Educational Research, 77*(1), 81–112.

Kluger, A. N., & DeNisi, A. (1996). The effects of feedback interventions on performance. *Psychological Bulletin, 119*(2), 254–284.

CHAPTER TWENTY-TWO

Building a Sustainable Learning System

Key Question

What keeps a learning system working through the hardest stretches?

Core Idea

A durable system keeps producing useful information and workable adjustments even when conditions do not cooperate.

Example Scenario

Falling behind in medical training rarely begins with one bad study session. More often, it begins when a learning system depends on conditions that medical training cannot reliably provide.

Aisha builds a detailed schedule and follows it for two weeks. Then a demanding rotation disrupts sleep, commute time, and attention, and restarting feels heavier than the original work. Another student studies well when rested but loses the thread after several nights of poor sleep. A third misses an exam question, then carries that result into the next block until every uncertain answer feels like evidence of a larger problem.

The situations look different. The underlying problem is often similar. The system was built for stable capacity, predictable time, and clean feedback. Medical training rarely provides those for long.

Closing the Loop

Feedback that is received but not converted rarely changes anything. The step that makes it count is turning it into a single next action, such as next time I lead with the assessment, so the information reaches the next attempt (Hattie & Timperley, 2007). Feedback answers how am I doing. The loop only closes when it also answers where to next.

Two habits keep the loop running. The first is generating your own feedback before seeking others': predict your question-bank score before revealing it and treat the gap as data about calibration instead of a grade (Butler & Winne, 1995). The second is keeping a short feedback log, so scattered comments become a trend, which connects to the self-doubt chapter's point that trends are steadier evidence than whichever impression is loudest today.

Feedback also has to stay usable. Medical training produces constant data: exam scores, question banks, evaluations, comments from supervisors, comparisons with peers, and the quieter feedback of how studying feels from day to day.

The trouble is not a lack of information. It is that the information often arrives under emotional load.

A practice score can feel like a prediction. A difficult evaluation can feel like a definition. A bad week can feel like a trend before there is enough evidence to call it one. When feedback becomes fused with identity, it becomes harder to use.

Feedback works better when it stays attached to the next adjustment. What pattern appeared? What condition contributed? What can change in the next study cycle?

A missed question might point toward more retrieval. A string of similar misses might point toward comparison work between diagnoses. Repeated trouble starting might point toward a task that is too vague. Poor performance after several depleted days might point toward capacity, not strategy alone.

The adjustment does not have to be large. In medical training, small changes are often more durable because they survive interruptions.

Decide the first task before stopping for the night. Limit the number of open resources. Use missed questions to identify mechanisms, not only topics. Return to material after a delay. Build in some retrieval before more review. Shrink the task when restarting feels too expensive.

These changes are not dramatic. They reduce friction where friction tends to accumulate.

Options Menu

Feedback only helps once it reaches the next attempt. Reach for whichever fits:

- **Turn feedback into one action.** Convert each piece into a single change for next time, not a note to feel. It is less than it seems you should do, and it is the part that reaches the next attempt (Hattie & Timperley, 2007).

- **Grade yourself first.** Predict the result before you see it, then read the gap as calibration data. It exposes a miss you would rather not see, and it is where accuracy comes from.

The Minimum Viable Day

Some days will not support a full study load, and the goal on those days is to keep the system running instead of matching a normal target. A Minimum Viable Day is the smallest defined unit of work that still counts as keeping up, decided in advance so a depleted evening does not turn into a lost one. It might be ten targeted retrieval attempts, a review of the questions missed earlier in the week, and choosing tomorrow's first task. It will not be four hours of dense new material across three resources. The point is continuity: a small day that happens preserves momentum that a perfect day skipped does not.

Also in the Field Manual, under Energy-State Tools.

The system also has to adapt as training changes. A method that works during a structured preclinical block may not work during a rotation with early mornings and fragmented time. A schedule that works during one month may fail during another. A resource that helps with recall may not be enough for clinical reasoning.

The old system was not wrong. The conditions changed.

The useful question becomes: what does this phase of training require from the system now?

Sometimes the answer is more retrieval. Sometimes it is better spacing. Sometimes it is less resource switching. Sometimes it is more recovery. Sometimes it is a narrower task, a clearer starting point, or a different way of reading feedback.

Adaptation is not a sign that the system failed. It is the maintenance work that keeps the system aligned with the conditions in front of you.

What ties these moves together is a cycle that self-regulated learners run more or less continuously: plan an approach, monitor how it is going, reflect on what the results show, and adjust before the next attempt (Zimmerman, 2002). Retrieval, calibration, recovery audits, and failure reviews are all instances of the same loop. The system this chapter describes is that loop, run on conditions that keep changing.

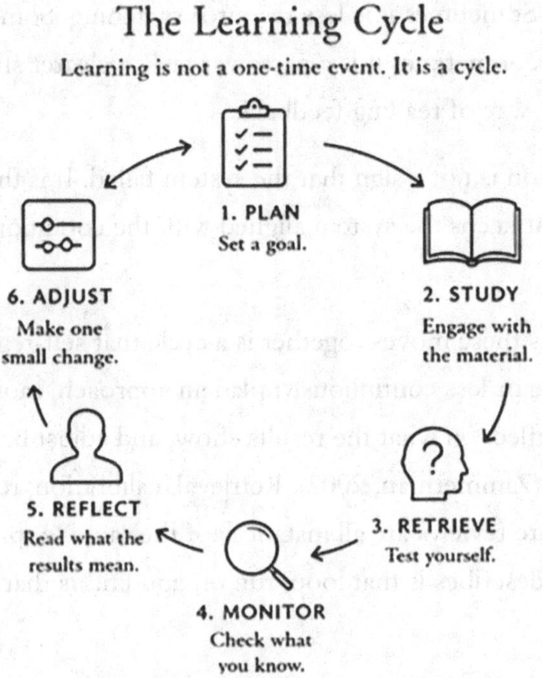

Figure 6. Self-regulated learning is a continuous cycle of planning, studying, retrieving, monitoring, reflecting, and adjusting. Small, deliberate adjustments accumulate into stronger learning over time.

The Regrouping Plan

After a disruption—a failed exam, a rotation that breaks your schedule, or a stretch of depleted days—the instinct is either to push harder or to rebuild the whole system from scratch. A regrouping plan is the middle path: a short, deliberate reset that keeps what still works and changes one thing.

Name the pattern across the recent stretch instead of the single worst moment. Identify the condition most likely driving it: load, access, strategy, emotion, recovery, or systems. Choose one change that fits that condition, small enough to survive the next interruption. Then run a normal cycle and read what happens.

Regrouping is the maintenance that keeps a system aligned with conditions that keep changing.

Also in the Field Manual, under Energy-State Tools.

Looking Through Longer Windows

Medical students often evaluate themselves through short windows: one exam, one week, one block, one rotation. Those windows matter, but they are incomplete. Learning usually develops across longer intervals than confidence does. Confidence can rise or fall quickly.

Competence often changes more gradually.

That mismatch can make progress hard to see.

A student may feel worse during retrieval practice while learning more. A student may feel better during review while leaving access undertrained. A student may feel behind after a difficult week while still building the system that will carry the next month.

The question is not whether every signal feels good. It is whether the system keeps producing useful information and workable adjustments.

- Can you test access?
- Can you interpret mistakes specifically?
- Can you notice when recovery is limiting capacity?
- Can you use feedback without turning it into a verdict?

- Can you adjust the task when the conditions change?

These are the habits that make learning more durable over time.

Closing the Book

The book began with a different way to read academic struggle. When studying stops working, the most useful question is usually not what is wrong with the student. A better question is what is happening in the learning system.

That question remains useful because the answer will keep changing.

Sometimes the problem will be load. Sometimes it will be retrieval. Sometimes it will be fatigue, anxiety, avoidance, comparison, feedback, or a task that has become too vague to enter. The work is to identify the mechanism closely enough that the next response fits the actual problem.

Medical training will continue to create difficult days. There will be missed questions, interrupted plans, uneven weeks, and moments when knowledge does not arrive on command.

A sustainable learning system is not one that prevents all of that. What it gives you is steadier: a way to keep learning while the hard weeks happen, and a way to read them as information, not a verdict. Across the length of training, that is what carries you.

Recap

What to hold onto for the long arc:

- **Studying is a system**, and its parts—load, access, strategy, emotion, recovery, and the systems you learn inside—interact rather than fail in isolation.
- Retrieval tests access, and calibration keeps the reading of a mistake specific.
- Recovery sets the capacity the rest of the system runs on.
- Feedback stays useful when it stays attached to the next small adjustment.
- A durable system keeps producing useful information and workable changes even through hard weeks.

References

Butler, D. L., & Winne, P. H. (1995). Feedback and self-regulated learning: A theoretical synthesis. *Review of Educational Research, 65*(3), 245–281.

Hattie, J., & Timperley, H. (2007). The power of feedback. *Review of Educational Research, 77*(1), 81–112.

Zimmerman, B. J. (2002). Becoming a self-regulated learner: An overview. *Theory Into Practice, 41*(2), 64–70.

Field Manual

The Study Systems

The chapters explain why studying behaves the way it does. These pages are for the part that comes after understanding: the ordinary work of planning a week, running a session, and turning a pile of missed questions into a short list of next moves.

This is not a planner, a schedule, or a single right way to study. Each system below is small, repeatable, and built from the same six conditions the book has used throughout: load, access, strategy, emotion, recovery, and the systems you learn inside. Use one when you need it, then close the book and return to the work.

Find the system that matches what you are doing:

Running on empty → *Energy-State Tools*

If you are not sure where to begin, let the problem decide. A week needs a map. A study block needs a shape. A missed question needs a diagnosis. Too many resources need a limit.

A few common situations have a quick version here and a fuller one in the first book:

If you are behind: do not try to repay every missed hour. Choose one current task, one repair task, and one question block, and re-enter there.

If capacity is low: run the minimum: a short retrieval block, one small set of misses reviewed, and tomorrow's first task written down.

After a hard exam: in the first raw hours, do not autopsy it while flooded. Steady yourself first, then come back to these systems.

Each of these connects to a chapter in this book: recovery and the minimum day to Chapter Fifteen, and the first hours after a hard result to Chapter Twenty-One. Use the quick form to keep moving, and turn to the chapter when you have room.

The Weekly Map

A container for the week, built once, so Sunday night is not spent rebuilding your life from scratch.

Use This For

Turning a week of lectures, deadlines, and question targets into a plan you can run, with recovery protected rather than postponed to a quieter week that never quite arrives.

The Moves

1. List what is due and what is testable this week. Separate the two. They are not the same, and confusing them is how low-yield work crowds out high-yield work.

2. Mark what needs understanding first and what needs retrieval practice. Put the understanding-first material early in the week, while attention is freshest.

3. Place your question blocks before anything else competes for the time. Decide how many, and on which days.

4. Protect one real recovery window, and write it in before the rest of the week fills the space around it.

5. Name the minimum version of the week: the two or three things that still happen even on a week that breaks.

6. Leave one block empty. The week will need it, and a plan with no slack shatters on contact.

How You Know It Is Working

You sit down most days already knowing the first task, and one bad day does not take the whole week down with it.

When It Breaks

If you are rebuilding the map every morning, it is too detailed. Plan in blocks, not hours, and let the blocks hold loosely.

Keep in Mind

The map is a container, not a contract. A plan you can adjust beats a plan you abandon.

See also: Chapter Fifteen, for the days when even the minimum is too much.

The Study Session

A shape for a single block of study time, so the hour produces access and not just activity.

Use This For

Structuring ordinary study time when you have a block and the material in front of you, and you want to leave with something you can retrieve, not only something you have seen.

The Moves

1. Name the target. One topic or one skill for this block, written down where you can see it.

2. Orient. Read or review just enough to hold the shape of the material. Resist letting this step quietly become the whole session.

3. Engage. Work the material actively: explain it, solve with it, build something from it. This is the longest stretch.

4. Retrieve. Close the material and produce it from memory, on paper or aloud. This is the step that builds access, and the one most often skipped.

5. Check. Look at what you missed, and name the kind of miss, not only the fact. (See Reading a Missed Question.)

6. Decide the next action and write it down before you stop. Tomorrow's session starts where this one ends.

Shorter version: target, engage, retrieve, check, decide next. The retrieve step is the one that cannot be cut.

How You Know It Is Working

By the end you can produce the material with the book closed, not only recognize it with the book open.

When It Breaks

If the block keeps becoming all orienting and no retrieval, shrink the target. A smaller target retrieved beats a larger one only reviewed.

Keep in Mind

Time in the chair is not the product. Access is the product, and the retrieve step is where one becomes the other.

Reading a Missed Question

A way to turn a block of missed questions into a short list of specific next moves, instead of a grade.

Use This For

Every missed or guessed question in a practice block. The score tells you how it went. The misses tell you what to change.

The Moves

1. For each miss, resist reading the explanation and moving on. First, name the kind of miss.

2. Sort it into one of these:

Knowledge: you never learned it.

Retrieval: you knew it but could not produce it without the options.

Discrimination: you narrowed it to two and chose wrong.

Application: you knew the fact but not how to use it in the stem.

Stem reading: you answered the question you expected, not the one asked.

Conditions: you knew it, but you were tired or rattled and access dropped.

Overthinking: you had it, and talked yourself out of it.

3. Match the repair to the kind:

Knowledge: a brief, targeted read, not a whole-topic reread.

Retrieval: closed-book recall.

Discrimination: a short compare-and-contrast of the pair that fooled you.

Application: more questions in that format.

Stem reading: slow the read, and name what is being asked before looking at the options.

Conditions: adjust the conditions, not your estimate of your preparation.

Overthinking: a decision rule you trust under pressure.

4. Keep a short running log of the kinds, not the questions. The pattern across a week tells you more than any single miss.

How You Know It Is Working

A block of forty questions becomes a handful of specific moves, most of them smaller than the studying you were about to add.

When It Breaks

If every miss keeps landing in knowledge, look again. A retrieval gap answered with rereading feels productive and stays fragile.

Keep in Mind

A missed question is a report on where access broke, not a verdict on whether you belong here.

See also: Chapter Twenty-One, for the first hours after a hard block, before this is useful.

Choosing Resources

A rule for resource overload: one primary, one practice, one backup, and a high bar for switching.

Use This For

Deciding what to study from when there are more resources than any person could use, and the standing temptation is to add one more.

The Moves

1. For each course or block, choose one primary learning source. This is where you build understanding.

2. Choose one question source. This is where you test access.

3. Allow one backup reference, opened only when you are genuinely stuck on something specific.

4. Do not switch unless you can name the problem the switch solves. That everyone else uses it is not a problem the switch solves.

On Flashcards

Flashcards are one tool inside this system, not a parallel plan. They earn their place for facts, mechanisms, associations, criteria, and drug classes, the material that rewards quick, repeated retrieval. They are a poor fit for whole lectures, reasoning pathways, and concepts you have not yet understood. A few rules keep them honest: cards should ask you to produce, not recognize; make fewer, better cards; suspend low-value ones without guilt; tie new cards to questions you actually missed; and do not let keeping up with cards become the whole study plan.

How You Know It Is Working

You spend your study time learning rather than auditioning resources, and you can say why each of your three is on the list.

When It Breaks

If you are collecting resources faster than you are using them, the load itself is the problem. Close the new tab and run the three you have.

Keep in Mind

More resources feel like more preparation. Usually they are more load. Depth in a few beats contact with many.

The Learning Pipeline

A way to see where a topic actually is, because material matures in stages and does not arrive finished.

Use This For

Judging whether something is exam-ready, and knowing what kind of work moves it forward from where it actually sits.

The pipeline: exposure → understanding → retrieval → discrimination → durability → performance under pressure. Each stage is built by different work, and a topic is only as exam-ready as the last stage it has passed.

The Moves

1. Find where a topic actually sits on the pipeline above. Be honest about the difference: *I have seen it* is exposure, not mastery.

2. Do the work of the next stage, not the first. A topic already at retrieval does not need another reread. It needs a harder question or a delayed test.

3. Treat the later stages as the real target. Exams test discrimination, durability, and performance under pressure, not exposure.

How You Know It Is Working

You stop treating *I have seen it* as *I know it*, and your effort lands on the stage a topic is actually stuck at.

When It Breaks

If everything feels stuck at the bottom, you are probably rereading. Move one stage up: close the notes and try to produce it.

Keep in Mind

Seeing is the beginning of learning, not the end of it. This is also what the first book meant by access: what you can retrieve and use under real conditions, built one stage at a time.

Studying on Rotations

A loop for clinical learning, where the patients are the curriculum and study time is short and scattered.

Use This For

Keeping a study system alive during rotations, when the day is unpredictable and the old block-study rhythm no longer fits.

The Moves

1. Before the day, pick one focus: a patient, a problem, or a question you want to be able to answer by evening.

2. During the day, capture questions from real cases as they arise. One line each. Do not try to resolve them on the spot.

3. After the day, run one short retrieval block. Answer a few of the day's captured questions from memory, then check.

4. Each week, do a set of shelf-style questions and look at the patterns in what you missed.

5. Let the patients be memory anchors. What you saw attaches to what you read better than either does alone.

6. Study what you saw, then what you are likely to be tested on. The two overlap more than they appear to.

How You Know It Is Working

Cases and reading start reinforcing each other, and the shelf stops feeling like a separate universe from the wards.

When It Breaks

If there is no time to study, shrink the loop, not the consistency. One captured question and one retrieval beat a plan for two hours you will not get.

Keep in Mind

On rotations the curriculum walks in the door. The system is mostly catching what is already in front of you.

See also: Chapter Sixteen, for the experience of learning where others can see you.

Energy-State Tools

Two tools for the days when capacity, not knowledge, is the limiting condition.

The Minimum Viable Day

Use This For

Days that will not support a full study load, when the goal is to keep the system running instead of matching a normal target.

The Moves

1. Decide the minimum in advance: the smallest defined unit of work that still counts as keeping up, so a depleted evening does not turn into a lost one.

2. Keep it concrete. It might be ten targeted retrieval attempts, a review of the questions missed earlier in the week, and choosing tomorrow's first task.

When It Breaks

If the minimum quietly grows into four hours of dense new material across three resources, it has stopped being a minimum.

Keep in Mind

The point is continuity: a small day that happens preserves momentum that a perfect day skipped does not.

See also: Chapter Twenty-Two, where it sits inside the full learning system.

The Regrouping Plan

Use This For

After a disruption—a failed exam, a rotation that breaks your schedule, or a stretch of depleted days—when the instinct is either to push harder or to rebuild the whole system from scratch.

The Moves

1. Name the pattern across the recent stretch instead of the single worst moment.

2. Identify the condition most likely driving it: load, access, strategy, emotion, recovery, or systems.

3. Choose one change that fits that condition, small enough to survive the next interruption.

4. Run a normal cycle and read what happens.

When It Breaks

If the reset starts changing everything at once, it has become a rebuild instead of a regroup. A regrouping plan is the middle path: keep what still works and change one thing.

Keep in Mind

Regrouping is the maintenance that keeps a system aligned with conditions that keep changing.

See also: Chapter Twenty-Two, where it sits inside the full learning system.

A Note on Scope

These systems address how studying is built. If functioning keeps narrowing even when the study system improves, the issue may be wider than study strategy. The right next move is to widen the circle of support by reaching out to an advisor, a clinician, or your institution's resources. That is not a failure of discipline.

The point of these systems is not to make studying perfect. It is to keep the next move visible. Medical training will keep producing load, pressure, feedback, and uneven weeks. A study system does not remove those conditions. It gives you a way to keep learning inside them.

About the Author

Laura S. Woodward, Ph.D., works at the intersection of social psychology, student success, academic resilience, and medical education support. Her work focuses on how students learn, persist, and maintain confidence in demanding academic environments, particularly high-pressure settings such as medical training.

She draws on research in motivation, belonging, resilience, test anxiety, learning science, and student engagement, along with practical experience supporting learners through academic difficulty. Her approach emphasizes that students can meet high standards more effectively when they understand how learning, stress, recovery, feedback, and institutional systems interact.

She is the author of *Learning Under Pressure* and *Studying for Medical School*, both part of The Human Side of Medical Training series from Threshold Academic Press.

www.ingramcontent.com/pod-product-compliance
Lightning Source LLC
LaVergne TN
LVHW040517210926
848480LV00007BA/1493
* 9 7 9 8 9 9 4 7 9 2 7 4 2 *